EMOTIONAL WELL-BEING
AND MENTAL HEALTH

EMOTIONAL WELL-BEING AND MENTAL HEALTH

A GUIDE FOR COUNSELLORS AND PSYCHOTHERAPISTS

DIGBY TANTAM

FOREWORD BY
EMMY VAN DEURZEN

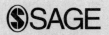

Los Angeles | London | New Delhi
Singapore | Washington DC

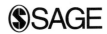

Los Angeles | London | New Delhi
Singapore | Washington DC

SAGE Publications Ltd
1 Oliver's Yard
55 City Road
London EC1Y 1SP

SAGE Publications Inc.
2455 Teller Road
Thousand Oaks, California 91320

SAGE Publications India Pvt Ltd
B 1/I 1 Mohan Cooperative Industrial Area
Mathura Road
New Delhi 110 044

SAGE Publications Asia-Pacific Pte Ltd
3 Church Street
#10–04 Samsung Hub
Singapore 049483

Editor: Kate Wharton
Assistant editor: Laura Walmsley
Production editor: Rachel Burrows
Marketing manager: Camille Richmond
Cover designer: Lisa Harper-Wells
Typeset by: C&M Digitals (P) Ltd, Chennai, India
Printed in India at Replika Press Pvt Ltd

© Digby Tantam 2014

First published 2014

Library of Congress Control Number: 2014930350

British Library Cataloguing in Publication data

A catalogue record for this book is available from the British Library

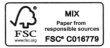

ISBN 978-1-4129-3108-3
ISBN 978-1-4129-3109-0 (pbk)

Contents

About the Author

Digby Tantam is Emeritus Professor at the University of Sheffield, an honorary visiting senior research fellow at the University of Cambridge and a director of the Septimus Group of companies.

He has been a psychiatrist in the NHS for most of his working life, and was the first Professor of Psychotherapy to be appointed to a UK University. He is married to Emmy van Deurzen, and they share the joys and occasional tribulations of their four children, and a love of the British countryside, where they live.

Foreword by Emmy van Deurzen

Many of us are preoccupied with the question of how to live our lives well. We know that it will involve knowing more about health, happiness and well-being but we get confused by the sheer contradictions between the contentions of authors in that field and might conclude it is best just not to think about it all too much and live from day to day.

This book tackles the age-old question of how to live in a direct and pragmatic manner. It seeks to find answers to existential questions by gathering the facts and making sense of them whilst weeding out the myths that still abound around these matters.

More books have been written about this subject than any of us could ever read. Digby Tantam's savvy summary of contemporary knowledge in this confusing field is concise and compelling in its clarity. From one chapter to the next he will guide you through the quagmire of fact and fantasy with the sure footedness of a highly experienced explorer and pathfinder.

Reading this book may therefore save you much trouble in your search for an authoritative text on the subject of well-being. It cuts right across the many different approaches to the science of happiness and gives you access to the different perspectives and angles that have evolved over the years. It summarizes the findings of philosophers, health economists, positive psychologists, health workers, politicians, religions and psychotherapists, showing you how to compare and contrast these views and go beyond them so that you begin to get a sense of what it all means.

When Digby and I started on a decade of happiness studies at the end of the nineties, as we co-directed the Centre for the Study of Conflict and Reconciliation at the University of Sheffield, we engaged in four funded projects to develop online masters programmes in existential psychotherapy in Europe together with many academic colleagues across the European Union. It soon became obvious that Digby's vision of existential investigation was uniquely challenging. It was always securely tethered in scientific research, careful observation and diligent reasoning and yet it was invariably given powerful wings by his unstoppable intellectual energy and commitment to philosophical enquiry and his capacity for synthetic meta-understanding.

This book, which was to be a handbook for the course, started out as a joint project, but I soon realized that I would be unable to keep up with the breadth, depth and speed of his investigation and analysis, as he filled the pages with great panache and certainty of purpose.

Much of his writing formed the basis of the online course we teach at the New School of Psychotherapy and Counselling on Health and Well Being, but for this manuscript he has augmented the original project and gone beyond it. It is a pleasure to be able to express my admiration for the excellence of his work as well as my gratitude for the steadiness and incisiveness of his exploration of these issues. Our collaboration has touched my own thinking greatly and he has stimulated me to conceive of existential psychology in a new and more contemporary way. Existential therapists have often had great insights into the philosophical aspects of human living, but they have often neglected to combine these insights with the lucidity of psychological, political or economic thinking. The mastery we can achieve when combining all these different methods, is displayed in this volume.

Digby weaves his canvas tightly, as he deftly pulls together strands derived from many different branches of investigation. You will find here a kaleidoscopic and erudite exploration of happiness, health and well-being, which will enlighten and enliven your thinking. If you follow these various threads and allow yourself to question your previous assumptions, you will start seeing the unfolding of a new canvas on which to redraw your own therapeutic practice as well as the way in which you are living.

1

Mapping the Territory: The Philosopher's Viewpoint – Living Well

Happiness and health are confusing. We all want them, but how we achieve them and even how we know that we have achieved them is more mysterious the more we look at it. We can say, 'I didn't realize how happy I was' or 'I thought I was happy, but it was all false'. So we can be unaware of or even be deceived about happiness. Similarly, we can say of someone who dies suddenly, 'He always seemed so healthy, and now this'. So we can be deceived about health, too.

> When it comes to saying in what happiness consists, opinions differ, and the account given by the generality of mankind is not at all like that given by the philosophers. The masses take it to be something plain and tangible, like pleasure or money or social standing. Some maintain that it is one of these, some that it is another, and the same man will change his opinion about it more than once. When he has caught an illness he will say that it is health, and when he is hard up he will say that it is money.

Aristotle caught this in his opening to the *Nicomachean Ethics*, and much of this chapter will be influenced by Aristotle's perspectives, and what more modern philosophers have made of them. As Aristotle also indicates in this quote, he did not think that health was a philosophically complex issue, unlike happiness. He, and other ancient philosophers, considered that it was a good, like money. You either had it or you did not. You knew when you did not, because as Aristotle writes, you had then 'caught an illness'. Ill health, like being wounded in battle, disabled, or losing all of your money, were the consequences of luck or the malign influence of the gods. Aristotle did accept that all of these things, and more unfortunate accidents besides, had a major impact on health. But he did not consider them as being under a person's control. They could not be aims, in the sense that happiness could be. Juvenal's tenth satire summarizes Aristotle's and his successor's opinions when he writes that we should pray for a healthy mind in a healthy body, and we should ask the gods to give us a stout heart that makes us uncaring about how long we live. All that a person can aspire to do, he concludes, is to live a virtuous life.

What virtue consists of continues to preoccupy us, and Aristotle is as relevant now as he was to the ancient world when considering what we should aim for. We continue to use lots of related but overlapping words for what we consider to be the aim of our lives. These include 'good luck' or being free of bad things happening to us; being free of pain; having as much pleasure as possible; being positively rewarded as often and as intensely as possible; experiencing well-being; living well; being satisfied with life; being well-regarded in our lives and after our deaths; and living forever in paradise. Each of these terms will come up in later chapters. They form a kind of sequence, from the most immediate satisfaction to the most long-term – indeed to a satisfaction that we can never experience in life but look forward to in death.

Health is conspicuously missing from this list. This is because it has not really been important in either ethics or politics – the two branches of philosophy to which happiness studies belonged, according to Aristotle – until quite recently, when modern medical science developed. Nowadays we recognize that our actions can increase our future risk of poor health; that our actions in relationship with others can affect another person's mental health; and that our actions as citizens can create policies that increase or decrease social inequities that directly affect mental and physical health. Because of the relative recency of these ideas, the ethics and politics of health have not been integrated into personal morality as deeply as the kind of question that the ancients were asking – questions like 'What does it mean to be a good person?' Most of us probably worry about whether we should eat as many cakes as we do, or whether contributing to a private health insurance scheme damages the health services available to people less well off, but we do not wake up asking ourselves these questions, with our hearts in our mouths. The 3.00 am kind of thought is much more likely to be: 'Did I do right? Am I a much worse person than I would like to think? What will people think of me?' These are the questions that I deal with in this chapter, but I will return to health philosophy in the next chapter, on public health and the health economist (Chapter 2), and in the chapter on the politician's viewpoint (Chapter 5).

Feeling good

There is no definite feeling that goes with being healthy, but there is a feeling of happiness. Not only that but the same things that Aristotle thought made people happy – getting something we want and so feeling pleasure, being rewarded and feeling pleasure at that, recovering from some illness or adversity, or feeling proud of our social status – still make people happy. So it is, perhaps, surprising that we can be as unclear about it as Aristotle was. It didn't seem so difficult when we were children. A Christmas morning with a stack of good presents seemed enough to give a lot of pleasure, and make one feel happy. But perhaps even that is an over-simplification of the kind that adults often make about their own childhoods. One of the few surveys of children (Chaplin, 2009) involved asking 300 children what made them happy. The children's responses were grouped by the interviewers into five categories: people and pets, sports, academic achievements, material possessions (not their own, mainly, but those of their parents), and hobbies. There was no instance of even the youngest child saying 'Eating my favourite ice-cream all day would make me happy'. Whether this reflects the interviewers' values, that this would not really be happiness, or whether it reflected the children's own values, vicariously adopting their parents' values, is not clear. What is clear is that, even in childhood, happiness is not purely based on pleasure.

One way that parents direct their children's desire for pleasure is by detaching pleasure from the moment, and summing it over the future instead. 'If you keep eating all those sweet things', a mother might say, 'your teeth will get really bad and you'll have to go to the dentist lots; you'll get fat and the other kids will call you names; and you'll probably end up being ill'. She might go on to say, 'But if you keep ice-cream as a special treat, it will taste all the better when you do have it'. Prudence shapes our ideas of what we have to do to be happy – that is, to be in a continuing state of happiness – and reduces the value of momentary pleasure.

We can only exercise prudence if we know what the future holds, however, and of course we cannot know, but we can turn to wise people who sometimes claim to do so.

The priestly view

Some of the earliest recorded recipes for happiness leave the whole matter to God or the gods. The gods, it is assumed, know what is good for people, and sooner or later they will provide it, in the shape of the Elysian fields, or paradise or heaven (many of us still adopt this providential approach to our health). Priests can interpret what the gods want, and can also provide the appropriate ceremonials, prescribed activities and rules of conduct that will make the god(s) happy and he or she will, in turn, make the worshipper happy – in the long run, at least. It is easy to see that gods are not just there to make people happy: if they were, there would be a lot less suffering in the world. They are also there to make people good (or so the priests tell us). So the gods also devise unpleasant experiences as tests of the faithful. Extended accounts of tests like this can be found in many religions' holy books and in folk-tales: examples include the book of Job, the Ramayana, the Journey to the West and the labours of Hercules. Happiness, according to the priests, thus consists in doing what will please the gods.

This strategy depends on having gods that are just, and who repay their worshippers for their worship. But there are plenty of theologies, perhaps especially in Asia and Africa, that have gods that are unjust, mischievous or even malignant. Some cosmogonies, like Manicheanism, believe that the world in which we live has been created by a malignant demon and not a god at all. Good people may therefore be punished and evil people rewarded. Many of the Mesopotamian city states seem to have such a cosmogony. It is described in one of the world's earliest known stories, now known as the epic of Gilgamesh which dates from 2150–2000 BCE, and describes the life of a possibly existent king of Uruk (now Iraq), Bilgamesh. Bilgamesh, or Gilgamesh as he is known in the later and fuller Akkadian version, was a hedonist. He took the virginity of every bride in his kingdom by *droit de seigneur*. Gilgamesh lived at a time when there was constant war between the city states of Mesopotamia, leading to cities being sacked, and when even militarily successful cities could be destroyed by flooding. The Epic of Gilgamesh makes reference to a great flood in the eastern Mediterranean that is thought by some to be the same flood mentioned in the Greek myth about Deucalion and the Hebrew myth about Noah. In Mesopotamia, the flood was put down to strife between the gods: Marduk destroyed earlier gods (perhaps the gods of other city states) and made people out of the fragments, but Enlil was angry and tried to get back at Marduk by raising the flood to destroy mankind, Marduk's creation.

Gilgamesh's hedonism is perhaps unsurprising in such a chaotic world, and his abuse of power is what we would expect – although perhaps wrongly – of a primitive ruler. However, the gods did not approve and sent an agent, Enkidu, to oppose Gilgamesh. Enkidu needed a bit of humanizing, duly provided by a temple prostitute, but is then ready to oppose Gilgamesh. They became fast friends, and Gilgamesh abandoned the brides to go on a quest with Enkidu. They succeeded in it, but the goddess Ishtar was so impressed that she wanted to make Gilgamesh her consort. He knew that Ishtar, the goddess of fertility, killed her consort every year, just when the wheat is harvested. So he refused and she, miffed, sent a bull to ravage Uruk (Iraq). Gilgamesh and Enkidu killed it, but Ishtar then killed Enkidu – and Gilgamesh's quest became a quest for immortality. He asked the way of another goddess, Siduri, the goddess of alcohol. She told him just to have a good time, and not bother about life and death, which are issues for the gods.

The epic of Gilgamesh illustrates the evolution of human ideas about gods, but also illustrates a shift in values linked to this. Perhaps the invention of writing played a role, as rulers' actions have, from that time, been recalled and commented on by subsequent generations. Rulers started to think about accountability, and could no longer simply use their power to pursue their own personal pleasure. They started to value using their power to protect the weak (killing the divine bull that ravaged Uruk) and pursue transcendent values (overcoming death). Intoxication plays an important role in the story, too, as a means for the gods to keep the rulers content to be pleasure seekers, and thereby stop them trespassing on to divine territory.

Another point illustrated by the Gilgamesh story is that society needs to regulate the powerful if they are not to become too damaging. Hobbes thought that this was achieved by a social contract, but the Gilgamesh story suggests that it is the temple that does it, by formulating the rules that will allow immortality, in paradise.

The philosopher's perspective

The ancient Greek philosophers, on whose work Western philosophy is still largely based, seem to have had little faith in an after-life, but did think that it was possible to nearly reach complete happiness in this life. Their attitude to suffering was curiously fatalistic. The gods, they thought, were no more moral than other beings and could easily make people suffer in the interests of their own jealousies and rivalries, as indeed the Gilgamesh story conveys. The only kind of human behaviour that the gods would not tolerate was hubris: the attempt of a human being to become god-like, and therefore a rival to themselves. Even this notion, though, was relaxed and heroic humans could be turned into stars and other immortal, if ineffectual, entities.

Greek philosophy was the product of a lucky few full citizens of Greek cities. They were protected from the sudden reversals of fate that influenced Mesopotamian cultures that were developed on flood plains. They could, and did, discount everyday pain and suffering from disease or overwork, or the hopelessness of leading a life controlled by other people. Their focus was on how people could rule themselves.

Aristotle is the Greek philosopher who is most influential in modern day happiness studies. Aristotle (384–322 BCE) was born and brought up as an Athenian citizen in the Chalcis peninsula. His father was physician to the King of Macedon, Amyntas. Aristotle moved to Athens to study in Plato's Academy, getting there some 15 years after Socrates had been executed. He stayed there until Plato died some 20 years later, and was then headhunted to be tutor to Amyntas's grandson, Prince Alexander of Macedon (later to be known as Alexander the Great). When Alexander was 16, Aristotle returned to Athens and formed his own philosophical school, the Lyceum.

Like that of Master Kong (Confucius), a retired chief police officer in a small Chinese kingdom, Aristotle's philosophy was directed at warriors, the up-and-coming aristocracy, rather than at priests. The Rig Veda, dating to the early iron age, and possibly originating in the Indus valley civilization, seems to have been similarly targeted at this new group of powerful members of civilized societies. It refers to the importance of honour to well-being. This is more thoroughly worked out in a tale of dynastic succession, the Mahabharata, written in the 5th century BCE and therefore roughly contemporaneous with Socrates. It chronicles the struggle between brothers to be able to perform the horse sacrifice reserved for kings. The Mahabharata includes one of the most famous Upanishads, the Bhagavad Gita, which sets out the correct means for a person to achieve well-being. It is especially relevant to the various ways that rta, or rightness, and the rules or dharma that typify rta, apply to kings and warriors. In fact, the Sanskrit word rta is the origin of the English word 'right', the Greek word 'arete' and probably the name of the god of battles, Ares. Arete in Greek originally meant excellence, presumably with something of the sense of 'rightness about it' (in Yorkshire, 'right' is still used in this sense, for example something that is excellent is 'right good').

Socrates was a friend of the famous Athenian mercenary captain Xenophon, with whom Socrates had served in a famous campaign in the Middle East. Socrates was a pugnacious character, as well as being an ex-soldier. One of the grounds for Socrates' execution was that he did not believe in the gods. He argued that living well would not just result in a person being given a place in heaven – he may not have even believed in heaven – but lasting happiness, which Socrates termed eudaimonia (we would probably now call this life satisfaction although it means, literally, good spirits). The key to this was to make the right choices. This is illustrated in the parable of the choice of Herakles, formulated by another friend, the sophist Prodikos. In this parable, Herakles was out walking and came to a crossroads. Two women stood there. Prodikos' description is lost, but this is how Xenophon, who had heard Prodikos' lecture, described one of the women: she was sluttish in her dress and manner but introduced herself as pleasure or happiness, although some knew her as Kakia (badness or vice). She says:

Herakles, I see that you are in doubt which path to take towards life. Make me your friend; follow me, and I will lead you along the pleasantest and easiest road. You shall taste all the sweets of life; and hardship you shall never know. First, of wars and worries you shall not think, but shall ever be considering what choice food or drink you can find, what sight or sound will delight you, what touch or perfume; what tender love can give you most joy, what bed the softest slumbers; and how to come by all these pleasures with least trouble. And should there arise misgiving that lack of means may stint your enjoyments, never fear that I may lead you into winning them by toil and anguish of body and soul. Nay; you shall have the fruits of others' toil, and refrain from nothing that can bring you gain. For to my companions I give authority to pluck advantage where they will. (Marchant, 1923; this translation is taken from the Marchant edition and translation of Xenophon's Memorabilia, book 2, chapter 1, section 12)

Xenophon goes on to describe the argument between two influential Greek philosophers of happiness over the interpretation of this parable. Socrates argued for arete and against vice, as can be inferred from the slanted way that Xenophon and his Victorian translator Marchant (Xenophon, Memorabilia 2.1.21) set the parable out. Another, African, philosopher, Aristippus, argued for pleasure, as I will discuss below.

Herakles' choice is cleverly constructed. It is realistic in that young, physical men like Herakles are likely to be easily turned from the path of duty by a pretty ankle (although, for obvious reasons, Xenophon took care not to portary Kakia as pretty), and that is a bugbear for military commanders (Aristotle wrote in his Ethics that young men were not 'fit students of moral philosophy', perhaps for this reason). But it presents moral choices in a skewed fashion. Had Herakles been starving, and had he to choose between an ignoble animal like a pig that he could run down and kill, or a noble animal like a stag whose hunt would give him glory, but likely no dinner, we would think badly of him if he chose the stag. Aristotle defined 'good' in the *Nicomachean Ethics* as that which all things aim at, and all things aim at survival. Had Herakles deliberated about his decision, both pig and stag would have run away. Had he told himself that he should consult his reason, and not his stomach, ditto. Had he said, 'I will not be like an animal', but will set aside my immediate desire in favour of a higher goal, he would have died of starvation. So most of us would think that a starving Herakles was right to give in to bodily sensation, and impulsively and unreasoningly so, focusing on immediate satisfaction rather than long-term glory. It was good that he did so.

A criticism of the notion of good desire just put forward might be that only some desires are necessities. Hunger prompts animals to feed and, without food, they would die. Sexual desire prompts copulation, and without copulation the species would die out. But very few instances of copulation are required to maintain the species. Sexual desire may also provoke people, and other primates, to non-reproductive sexual activity (here I leave out the much more complex relationship of intercourse to procreation, the biological importance of sexual competition for genetic health and the survival function of sexuality's role in reconciliation). Most of the time, sexual desire is not driven by a biological need and no longer meets the definition of a 'good' in being something that all things aim at. But many people might consider that regular sex between loving partners, even without the possibility of reproduction, is a 'good', not least in that it gives one partner the opportunity to provide the gift of pleasure to another. However, I am anticipating the kind of objection that Aristippus made to

Socrates' pious attitude to sex, and I should wait until I introduce Aristippus more formally below.

Aristotle made 'arete' a key element in his formulation of eudaimonia, which is often nowadays translated as 'happiness' but literally means 'good spirits', in the sense that people might say that someone is fine-spirited. Socrates has Arete, the personification of arete, in telling Herakles that pleasure is short-lived and appetites get jaded. Aristotle makes a more principled argument. He argues that 'Every art and every inquiry, and similarly every action and pursuit, is thought to aim at some good; and for this reason the good has rightly been declared to be that at which all things aim' (first sentence, book 1 of the *Nicomachean Ethics*). This must have seemed all the more obvious to Aristotle as his name translates as 'good aim'. Aristotle goes on to discuss what is good. Lower-class people, he says, think that pleasure is good. More refined people think that honour is good. But one can be honoured when one is asleep, he noted, and anyway being honoured for one's arete is generally more desirable to people than being honoured for anything else; so, Aristotle concluded, the possession of arete is more important than honour. Aristotle thinks that arete is the satisfaction of a job well done. A particular job is part of a larger project. So, developing arete for all of the jobs in this wider project, and indeed in the project itself, must be more valued than doing a single job well. Each project can itself be subsumed into an even bigger project – living a life. So the arete, or skill with which one lives all aspects of one's life, is the greatest source of satisfaction. One of the important contributions to this skill is the acquisition of phronesis or practical wisdom.

It might seem obvious when one exercises a skill 'rightly'. One can look at one woman's dressmaking and see that she has done it excellently, or one man's digging in the garden and see that he has been sloppy. But it's much less clear what the criteria should be for more abstract tasks. Aristotle falls back on prior values, particularly nobility. Nobility is a set of values that we look for in warriors or rulers, but not so much in monks or dentists. So Aristotle's claim to be setting out universal values looks over-ambitious. Even so, many of his successors have sought to specify lists of values that will lead to life satisfaction, and they constitute one of the three main philosophical approaches to happiness and well-being. They are sometimes called objective list theorists, as opposed to hedonists, and desire satisfaction theorists.

Aristotle considers three objections to his idea that virtue is sufficient to lead to life satisfaction. The first is that misfortune makes people unhappy and feel less satisfied with their lives, which seems to undermine his notion that what a person does with their circumstances is the key to happiness. He brushes this off with the idea that 'when the going gets tough, the tough get going' or, rather, when nobility is hard pressed, then true nobility is expressed. Later, he admitted that some suffering is so extreme that it ruins life satisfaction: no one can be expected to be happy on the rack (the Stoics thought that they could). This is, therefore, a limit to his theory of happiness although others who follow Aristotle have not always conceded this.

A second objection is related. Only some people are in a situation, or have the character, or have been given the right parenting, to be 'noble'. Without this basic stuff of nobility, no amount of work on oneself (no amount of accumulated practical wisdom) will result in eudaimonia. Aristotle considers this and by implication restricts his theory to those people who are born to the right parents, and with the right advantages, and who, as a result, have acquired the right 'moral' virtues (David Hume called these 'passions') to direct their intellectual virtues of practical reason.

A final objection is that some people, despite seeing the path to virtue, fail to take it. They are incontinent or show 'akrasia'.

There may have been another reason that Aristotle opposed reason or virtue and pleasure. As we have seen, arete derives from the ethics taught to warriors who were almost entirely men, and the word may have even derived from the name of the male god of battles, Ares. Arete also means strength in Greek and virtue is derived from 'vis' meaning strength in Latin, itself derived from 'vir' meaning man. Socrates and Aristotle both taught men and fraternized with soldiers. Women were excluded from the Academy and the Lyceum. Few Greek women were recognized as wise in Athens or later, in its philosophical successor, Rome. They were either graces, or furies, like Medea, Clytamnestra or Socrates' wife, Xanthippe. Aristotle's version of happiness was 'manly' in the sense that 'manliness' became a virtue of the English public school. It was the result of struggle, of freeing oneself from urges and desires, and of companionship with other free individuals, who had won the right to have their needs met by others.

The values behind Aristotle's philosophy included the belief that men were superior to women and children, citizens to private individuals, or idiots, both to slaves, and Greeks to barbarians, i.e. Persians. Men were superior because they were the only group to be politically, i.e. publicly active, and this was rationalized by the notion that men were dominated by reason, and women by emotion. Emotions were linked to the body: this must have seemed obvious as bodily states such as being wounded, being pregnant, having a period, being ill are all associated with strong emotions. So Aristotle's culture not only opposed men and women, but also body and mind or soul, emotions and reason, and sometimes conflated each of these polarities into one: weak and strong.

Religious writers have agreed. The Iranian, Mani, thought that the body was evil and the mind was good (BeDuhn, 2000), pushing the argument further in favour of dualism. St Augustine, himself a Manichean before his conversion to Christianity, considered that the body was a source of temptation that had to be disciplined, and 'pleasures of the flesh' continue to be distrusted by many Christians who, like the followers of Opus Dei, may use self-wounding or 'mortification' as a means of obtaining goodness.

The perspective of the dispossessed

Persian culture was voluptuous and its men effeminate, so far as the Greeks were concerned. There was no recognition that the Persians could be virtuous except when they imitated the Greeks. Greek cities were separated by mountains or deep inlets and were often at war. The Persians built an enormous empire held together by good roads, and an excellent messenger service. Autonomy was a virtue to the Greeks, connectedness to the Persians. Women could rise to power in the Persian empire or in its remains: Cleopatra in Egypt and the legendary Sheba in Sudan are examples. The most famous

Greek woman to be recognized for her wisdom, Cassandra, lived in what is now Asia, in the far west of Turkey, and so was almost within the Persian empire. She was wise, and, like other Eastern women, she could foretell the future. But like a Greek woman, her prophecies fell on deaf ears (there were exceptions to this, of course, including the Pythia at Delphi, although here utterances were interpreted by male priests, and the queen of the Ionian state of Halicarnassus who commanded a fleet in the naval battle at Salamis that stopped Xerxes invasion of Greece) (an exception to this generalization is Artemisia). Iranian culture and the cultures that assimilated its values, the Sassanids, the Arabs and the Moors, the Turks and the Moghuls, placed a much higher value on pleasure, which resulted in a very different conception of happiness. This stressed connectedness or mergence over autonomy.

Wine was first developed in Turkey and spread from there into Europe, including into Greece. The use of wine became the basis of the cult of Dionysus or Bacchus, one of whose high points was a yearly orgy of drinking and, reputedly, sexual indulgence. Contemporary accounts of this are filtered through the dramatic requirements of the Greek theatre, but they suggest that Bacchic rites particularly involved women, often had a strong androphobic element and broke down social barriers amongst women. Women considered that they had been taken over by the divine, anarchic spirit of Dionysus: 'enthusiasm'. The Greeks seem to have considered the Bacchae in their revels something like French intellectuals thought of the Parisian rioters of the 1870s or we think of crowds of football hooligans now. Bacchic rites have not completely disappeared: modern versions include 'raves' and even drunk nights out in South Yorkshire (Bennett, J. personal communication). Enthusiasms have also been noted in the animal world, too, with monkeys and other mammals converging on trees whose fallen fruit has fermented, and showing apparent signs of inebriation once they have eaten it.

Enthusiasm is as much a kind of happiness as the practice of the skilled craftsman or the philosophical practice of contemplation (Aristotle's highest form of satisfaction). But it is associated with mergence rather than skill. Hinduism has strongly recognized mergence as a source of well-being. For example, the Bhagavata Purana claims that supreme happiness and true joyfulness follow from mergence with Brahman.

Drink stops people thinking clearly: it overpowers the reason that Aristotle thought was so essential to a person achieving arete. To return to Aristotle's illustrations from craftwork, the arete of a leather worker required a nice bit of leather to work on, and then the knowledge that comes from long practice to work it to the final product. The latter kind of practical knowledge, or phronesis, is what alcohol subverts. Drunk leather workers do not produce good bridles. Alcohol increases incontinence or akrasia: a lack of willingness to apply and follow through on practical reasoning. It also increases the risk of blunders in that reasoning.

Alcohol is not the only factor that adversely affects reasoning. Aristotle supposed, like many philosophers, that women, children and the lower classes are incontinent and therefore defective in reason. This is one reason that the ancients thought that women could not be allowed to vote, and why we still do not give the vote to children. The Bacchic rites would simply have reinforced this view.

However, Aristotle's idea that women are more incontinent than men does not fit with the facts. Men are generally more impulsive and unbridled. Men commit more crimes than women, are heavier users of alcohol and drugs and have a lower life expectancy (Y. Zheng & Cleveland, 2013). There are famous examples in literature of men being put to death for interrupting Bacchanals, but of course it is not possible to obtain accurate information about how dangerous they were, or whether they led to better or worse behaviour long term, or to greater or lesser happiness. Livy brought a case to the Roman Senate of violence and rape (Riedl, 2012) of a young man during a Roman Bacchanalia, but there is reason to suppose that this was politically motivated. Livy describes this particular Bacchanal in detail, confirming that it was organized by women, that women outnumbered men and that it particularly attracted people who were not Roman citizens. The modern equivalent of the Bacchanal, the rave, in which ecstasy usually replaces alcohol, is not associated with violence.

Bringing together a lot of men, for example in a football crowd, is associated with a heightened risk of violence. So this suggests that, contrary to Aristotle and subsequent male philosophers, women are less and not more likely to act out their passions, their emotions, than men, and that the Bacchanal is not primarily an excuse for lust, but provides the experience of mergence, referred to in the Bhagavata Purana (Anon, 2009). The followers of Dionysus or Brahman attribute the effect to the diminution of self-consciousness – just acting spontaneously or not thinking about oneself, as it is sometimes described.

Aristotle conceded that temperament extends 'autos' or self to include other people, for 'man is by nature adapted to a social existence', but when he starts to enumerate who should be included within the self – he mentions parents, children, wife, friends, and countrymen – he then realizes that there is a problem and notes that 'some limit must be fixed: for if one extends it to parents and descendants and friend's friends, there is no end to it'. But he does not see a solution: 'This point must be left however for further investigation', he writes.

Aristotle is here raising the issue of what Auguste Comte was later to term 'altruism' (vivre pour autrui): why we should take account of other people's happiness in our own. Aristotle tries to deal with it as an aspect of practical reason, but, as is obvious from the previous paragraph, he fails. Nor does practical reasoning explain the kind of enthusiastic joining with other people that characterized the Bacchanal or currently characterizes the rave. The love of a mother for her child is often cited as the most intense example of altruism, and some psychologists have suggested that women have a particular skill in, and disposition towards, this kind of fellow feeling. An alternative explanation is that we are emotionally linked to other people in an unreasoning, reflexive way. Hume called this sympathy, Schleiermacher shared subjectivity, Husserl intersubjectivity and Lipps and Stein 'Einfühlung', translated by Titchener as 'empathy'. I call it the 'interbrain' (Tantam, 2009). Empathy means that other people's emotions automatically impinge on our own, unless we make a conscious effort to cut them off. If we have empathy for someone, we cannot be fully happy if they are sad, or really sad if they are happy.

The perspective of the man or woman in the street

Xenophon was an officer, and his account of Socrates gives an officer's viewpoint. We would probably have considered him a bit of a toff nowadays, and Socrates a bit common. The latter's father was a stonemason, and he may have also worked as a mason before becoming a soldier. Plato's account of Socrates' views of happiness was a lot closer to Aristotle's views of what the vulgar thought: that one should take pleasure where one finds it. In the *Gorgias*, Socrates (Plato, 1959) indicates that pleasure is not necessarily bad, even if it is self-indulgent (he specifically mentions food, drink and sex) and only becomes bad, i.e. worth avoiding, if in the long run it leads to greater pain. However, he does also say that one has to be satisfied with just living out one's life as pleasantly as possible and with the minimum of pain. Not everyone will be satisfied.

Many people turn to pleasure without thinking that, in the long run, it may lead to pain: health awareness programmes often focus on this, enjoining us to 'Think...' about the consequences of whatever issue is current, such as sex without condoms. Clearly for Socrates, as for many of us, prudence seems an important requirement of happiness. Deferring pleasure in accordance with prudence requires self-control and psychological research has linked this to self-reported happiness (Hofmann et al., 2013).

If the future is likely to be short and uncertain, as Gilgamesh thought it might be, given the flooding that had wiped out Mesopotamian civilization, then it is prudent not to delay gratification but to take one's pleasure whilst you can. Suppose one had AIDS, and it had become resistant to all of the antivirals, one could see that it would make sense to spend one's last few months trying to have as much sex as possible, perhaps with as many people as possible, if one believed that pleasure can produce happiness. Most other people would, however, regard that as an act of desperation, rather than of a well-lived life. Nor would it be living well in the sense of taking other people into account, as promiscuous sex when one has HIV is likely to spread the virus to other people.

Socrates considers this kind of situation in the *Philebus* (21 a-d) when he asks Philebus if he would accept a life spent entirely in the enjoyment of the greatest pleasures (Plato, 1975). Philebus says that he would, but then asks Philebus to imagine living this life without thought, memory, knowledge and true belief. Without memory, Socrates pointed out, Philebus would not have the pleasure of recalling past pleasure, and without thought would not have the pleasure of anticipating future pleasure. Philebus agrees that he would not prefer a life of pure pleasure, without reason, thus opening the door for Aristotle's idea that reason itself can lead to happiness, not through pleasure but through satisfaction.

This is not entirely a knock-down argument. Philebus could have retorted that he wanted reason and memory precisely because they increased the opportunity for pleasure; that, at the end of the day, maximizing pleasure is what drives all animals, including people. This is the position of the hedonist, exemplified by Socrates' opponent in the discussion of the choice of Herakles, the Cyrenian and Aristippus the elder, and by the younger Epicurus.

Hedonists may seem uninterested in the difference between pleasure and happiness, but, as Philebus' discussion with Socrates indicates, they are not the same. Not all pleasures are associated with happiness. Aristotle cites the pleasure of recovering after an illness. One could say of this, 'I am happy to have survived' but if one were asked before getting ill, 'Would it make you happy to be ill in the near future?' the answer would obviously be 'no'. So hedonism is more than fatalism. Hedonists want to increase their pleasure as much as possible, and so choose a greater pleasure over a lesser, in this case the greater pleasure of having full health over the lesser pleasure of getting better from illness. Bringing choice into the situation makes it explicit that hedonists also make pleasure an aim and interpret the aim of having a happy life to mean having a maximally pleasurable life rather than a good life.

Most of us think of pleasure like Philebus. It involves food, drink or sex (one might add money to this, and perhaps, too, the exercise of power and control over other creatures).

Hedonists are therefore up against an existential problem: this kind of pleasure is nice but, like the proverbial Chinese meal, it's often not very satisfying. An hour after you've eaten, you feel hungry again. Having a lot of money often makes people want to have even more. In fact, biology is such (I will consider the evidence in a later chapter) that the more one indulges in this kind of pleasure – often called 'reward' in the biological sphere – the greater the tolerance one develops for it, the less pleasure given by the same level of reward, and the harder it is to regain the same heights of pleasure as previously.

The perspective of the egotist

Aristippus was a contemporary of Socrates. His daughter, Arete (an ironic choice of name on the part of her father, no doubt), and her son, Aristippus the younger, are collectively known as the Cyreniacs as they all lived in Cyrene, in modern-day Libya. They argued against quietism and for a kind of robust hedonism. Like the song-bird who sings on a glorious summer day, they thought that we should make the most of happy moments and allow our happy feelings to swell. However, they did accept the Epicurean argument that most people are not satisfied with feeling happy; most also want it to last as long as possible and, if it doesn't, most people feel disappointment, anger or regret. The Cyrenaics argued that this was a kind of faulty thinking. It's best to take happiness wherever and however you find it, without expecting it or believing that one has a right to it or that it will last forever. And when it does go, don't repine, but take steps to lead life so that one has the best chance to be happy again.

Aristippus had considerable self-confidence, which was probably not misplaced. There is a story about him being washed up in Rhodes, having lost all his belongings when the ship he was voyaging on foundered. He blithely walked into the city, into the gymnasium, got chatting to other people there, who liked his company and gave him a helping hand, and within a short while he was once again profiting from his advisory services (he was a paid professional philosopher or sophist) and on his way back to prosperity. He had the post-modern idea that all a person needed to get on was what they had between their ears. Little accurate is known about his life, or even about his philosophy, since the main sources wrote centuries after he lived. But he is also credited by these sources with actions that are less attractive, such as exposing his infant son because he was not wanted, or toadying to his regal sponsor, by cross-dressing and dancing.

The Cyreniacs shared with Pyrrho and other sceptics the idea that we never grasp the world as it is, but only as it is influenced by our perspective and our emotional dispositions. Pyrrho likely adopted this from Vedic or Buddhist philosophers that he encountered in India, whilst serving with Alexander's army. The Hindus and the Buddhists would have added that our emotional attachments can be put aside, to reveal the world as it is. The Cyreniacs rejected this: they believed that our sensuality is the only thing that we can really take to be real. Since past and future pleasures are only ghosts of our present feelings, then it is present pleasure or pain that is most real, and so only this present pleasure and not some future, vague and possibly misleading expectations of future pleasure that should concern us. The Cyrenians would therefore have agreed with one modern well-being guru, who advocates living in the now.

Cyrenian hedonism is often opposed on irrational grounds, for example that living to excess is always going to be bad for your health, or that indulgence is intrinsically wrong. But even so, our instincts do seem to be against it.

The Cyrenaics' belief that present pleasure is much stronger than past or future pleasure could be interpreted to justify the 'James Dean' effect or Maslow's (1968) peak experience.

The perspective of the undemanding

The other major branch of hedonism was first developed by Epicurus. He had a very systematic philosophy, although much of it has been lost. He thought of pleasure as being of two kinds: 'static' and 'kinetic'. Static pleasure was exemplified by eudaimonia, but Epicurus thought that life satisfaction was the result of achieving tranquillity and not perfecting arete. Tranquillity – ataraxia – can be achieved by overcoming anxiety, particularly what Epicurus thought was the main anxiety for most people – the fear of death. Kinetic pleasures arise, according to Epicurus, from satisfying desires, and are therefore always preceded by a want or need, a source of anxiety. Hence, kinetic pleasure is a perturbation that should be avoided if we aim for tranquillity. Epicurus therefore advocated a modest lifestyle, without any pleasure-seeking but with the aim of reducing anxiety of all kinds.

Epicureanism is a form of what is now called 'desire satisfaction theory': that life satisfaction comes about from getting what we want (and when we want it). There is a thread of hedonism in this, too, since it suggests that we will be more satisfied if we want more, and have those greater wants satisfied. But common sense tells us that this is exactly the situation Epicurus warned about when he argued that kinetic pleasure is always associated with a period of wanting, and therefore displeasure, and may even, summing over the period of wanting and then being satisfied, be a negative or unpleasant experience.

The Tathagata's Epicureanism

For Buddhists, as for Sakyamuni Buddha, the only kind of lasting happiness is the absence of suffering, and this can be achieved by the abolition of desire. This, Buddhists argue, need only pierce the veil of illusion that envelopes reality in our eyes, since it is the veil, and not the reality, that arouses our desire. The Buddha was perhaps thinking particularly of male sexual desire. The veil is, after all, one of the classic male turn-ons. A man may desire a skimpily dressed woman more than the same woman unclothed because he desires to undress her, not because he desires the woman for herself. In fact, some men find completely naked women disturbing rather than arousing. Inadequate clothing, no good for protection from the weather or from dust, but only designed for allurement, create the illusion that the woman has no needs of her own; that she exists only to please the man. The man relates not to the woman alone, but his emotional reaction is a generalized one to 'women in skimpy clothes'. So the desire is for, or so Buddhists think, the image of 'women in skimpy clothes' and not the woman herself. When our car breaks down in a storm on a lonely moor, we are frightened partly of our feelings about 'lonely moors', 'darkness' and 'storm'. We might even think that there is a malign presence that is working against us. We have to work to pierce this threatening haze over the situation, and start to think about this particular moor, this particular car and our particular resources. When we win a game of cards, we feel that luck is on our side. We may have to consciously remind ourselves that this instance of success has no bearing on the probability of future instances of success. We hope to propitiate the fate that is against us, or we imagine that luck has been drawn to us by some special personal attraction. So our peace of mind is disturbed by our efforts to propitiate, hold on to or otherwise secure a special relationship that we have invented.

The Buddha's argument is very similar to that of his approximate contemporary in Greece. Epicurus, like Buddha, created a kind of monastic following, although it petered out in the sceptical soil of Greece rather than flourishing as Buddhism did in the fertile soil of the land of the Vedas. Epicurus, whose name is ironically associated with the pleasures of the table, and whose philosophy of hedonism is, in another irony, applied nowadays to the pursuit of pleasure, was actually an advocate of self-denial. Like the Buddha, he argued that seeking pleasure meant wanting pleasure, and it was just a fact of life that wants are more often frustrated than satisfied. A happy life is one where the positive emotions outweigh the negative or, to put it another way, the hedonic balance is in the green and not the red. An obvious way to achieve that is to keep the number of things one wants to a minimum. As one tends to want to repeat a pleasurable experience, it is best to avoid pleasurable experiences. Epicurus did think that there were some pleasurable experiences that did not lead to disappointment, and these he called 'kastematic' although that has sometimes been translated as 'static'. They are the quiet pleasures that this section began with. The kinetic pleasures are the ones we get used to, want more of, for which we feel a growing need until we satiate them, and then we wonder why the pleasure seems so little after all – these pleasures are the ones that cause pain and in the long run push the hedonic balance into the red.

The public health perspective

It will have become obvious so far that happiness means different things to different people. One person may aim to be famous, another to be loved, another to be untroubled. One person may want pleasure now, another pleasure in a more lasting form in the future. An ascetic may want to feel hunger, knowing that they are gaining the satisfaction of self-denial.

Jeremy Bentham, as a Victorian philanthropist, wanted to benefit whole groups of people, and not just individuals (1876). It was, as Walter Benjamin noted, the age of the crowd. When Bentham considered how to do this, it must have seemed obvious that if you add all these different versions of happiness together, the differences average out. Whilst one could not be certain what an individual meant by happiness, if you asked 1000 or 10,000 people, a consensus would develop. It's the ballot box approach that we have adopted in democratic politics.

Jeremy Bentham was a social reformer first and a philosopher second. He assumed that the world should be a better place, and that this could be achieved if there was more happiness and less pain. Bentham's basic premise to his philosophy can be found in *An Introduction to the Principles of Morals and Legislation* (Bentham, 1876): 'Nature has placed mankind under the governance of two sovereign masters, pain and pleasure. It is for them alone to point out what we ought to do as well as to determine what we shall do' (1876: 225). Bentham never married, despite falling in love with all four daughters of his patron, Lord Lansdowne, but it would be wrong to conclude that in his private life he was a Benthamite. He wrote the following in one of his letters:

> Create all the happiness you are able to create: remove all the misery you are able to remove. Every day will allow you to add something to the pleasure of others, or to diminish something of their pains. And for every grain of enjoyment you sow in the bosom of another, you shall find harvest in your own bosom; while every sorry which you pluck out from the thoughts and feelings of a fellow creature shall be replaced by beautiful peace and joy in the sanctuary of your soul. (Bentham in a birthday letter to a friend's young daughter, quoted in Layard, 2011: 235–236)

Like his fellow utilitarian, J. S. Mill, his heart was in the right place, even if he did not march in step with his peers. He thought that as dogs and horses were more intelligent than human babies they deserved at least as much consideration as babies. In the same rationalist spirit, he supported equal rights for women, the separation of church and state, the abolition of physical punishment for children, money lending, greater access to divorce, the decriminalization of homosexuality, the French revolution (but not the Terror), free trade and university entrance for Protestants who would not swear their commitment to the articles of the Church of England ('Dissenters'). He said that he took the principles of the 'greatest good for the greatest number' from the Unitarian – and therefore, Dissenting – chemist, Joseph Priestley, whose own support for the French revolution had led to his house and his chapel being attacked with fire bombs.

Although Bentham, in the passage quoted above, described two masters, one of pleasure and one of pain, he did not pursue their independence but treated them as partners who were so conjoined that pain could be considered a negative amount of pleasure. This is much the same step that the Cyreniacs took, and it suffers from the same inconsistency that their philosophy did, not least that people do not simply base their happiness on pleasure received. Happiness has an aspirational element. As Aristotle said, it is a goal. Pleasure does not motivate us in the same way. This is demonstrated by some famous experiments by two psychologists, Kahneman and Tversky. They showed (Tversky & Kahneman, 1974) that simply adding the pleasure of an experience and subtracting its pain does not predict motivation, as well as a more complicated calculus that takes account of factors like recency and risk. For example, people prefer to repeat the experience of having their hand in very cold water (just above 14°C) for a minute, leaving it there for a further 30 seconds whilst the water is very slightly warm, than to repeat having their hand in very cold water (again, just above 14°C) for a minute, and then removing it immediately. The former provides less pleasure but also makes people less unhappy and so is preferred. Kahneman and Tversky argue that a calculation about which situations make us more or less happy is not based on the sum of the pleasure or pain of an experience, but is based on our feelings at the peak of the experience averaged with our feelings at the end of the experience.

Bentham was focusing on averages, and particularly group averages. He devised a metric, the felicific calculus that he thought would enable a calculation of the amount of pleasure an event would produce, taking account of such factors as how long the pleasure would last, how strong the sensation was, how likely it was that it would be followed by pain, and so on. Probably no one used the 'felicific calculus' to work out how to act but it has proved a very useful tool to consider how the average man, or group, should act when coupled with Bentham's other idea that the best action is the one that provides the greatest good to the greatest number.

Bentham's calculus works much better as a means of calculating the balance of pleasure and pain that many people feel about an experience because, like large-scale surveys or polls, the effect of individual variation becomes less and less important as the sample gets larger. In fact, so consistent does the opinion of masses of people become that Bentham seems to have forgotten that pleasure and pain are values that individuals place on things, and spoke about them as if they were caused by some property of the things themselves. He called this property a 'utility' (Bentham, 1876), defined as 'that property in any object, whereby it tends to produce benefit, advantage, pleasure, good, or happiness … or … to prevent the happening of mischief, pain, evil, or unhappiness'. (ibid., p. 2)

Bentham's derivation of a common property that would explain any pleasure and any pain seems a brilliant stroke in one way, but it seems weird in another. After all, it's not the property of an object to produce pain or happiness, rather it's our reaction to it. Handing someone a very hot piece of metal might cause pain, and that would be due to a property of the metal, i.e. its heat. But handing a person a photograph of their wife who was shortly due back from a long trip abroad might well cause pleasurable anticipation, or the pain of separation, but hand the same photo to a stranger and it is unlikely that it will cause any strong feeling. The pleasure or pain is not a property of the photograph, but a consequence of our reaction to it. This reaction will not be a fixed quality: not like the heat of the metal in the first example, but like the photo, to which the husband's reaction is likely to be different on the day after his wife has left to that on the day that she is due back.

His assumption that utility resides in the object rather than in its evaluation is precisely the kind of error that critics think that quantitative researchers make: that they ignore the meaning of what they study. As I showed in the discussion of democracy, individual meaning is not so relevant for policy making which has to apply to many different individuals for whom meaning tends to average out. Bentham's approach appeals much more to the rulers than the ruled.

Meaning is relevant though for most of us having to make a decision for ourselves or our loved ones. A health organization might be willing to introduce a new drug for cancer even if a small proportion of people will die as a result of taking the drug – say, as an example, 0.5% – if the benefits of the drug are very great; 0.5%, 1 in 200, does not sound so great and as far as the vitality of the total population taking the drug is concerned, that has only been reduced to 199/200. But if I am considering taking the drug, my vitality is not going to be reduced by that amount: I will either survive or my vitality will be reduced to 0/200. I will die.

The gentleman's viewpoint

John Stuart Mill was a gentleman among philosophers. He mastered classical languages as a child and was familiar with the company of great men. He was in love with Harriet Taylor, and she with him, but they did not become a couple until 21 years later, after her husband had died. Harriet lived for seven years longer, and following her death in Avignon, Mill bought a house in the city, where she had died and he had spent half his year, to be near her grave. He, like David Hume, was fluent in French and, again like Hume, was influenced by French philosophy, particularly that of Comte. He believed in equality for women, the emancipation of slaves and respect for individual human rights. He was an active MP, trying to make the world a better place. He was also a Benthamite, except that he could not accept that any pleasure of equal value on Bentham's hedonic calculus was necessarily of equal value in ethical terms. Say that one person rated their pleasure in being present at a cockfight as X, and another their pleasure at reading Shakespeare as Y, and X = Y in the amount of pleasure received, X could not equal Y in value. Some pleasures were higher and some lower. Higher pleasures were moral or intellectual and lower pleasures more obviously appetitive. Higher pleasures were higher because people had to learn to appreciate them (for a modern restatement of this, see Grayling, 2007).

This is now a widely held view. It is one reason that there is strong support for the Arts Council to subsidize opera or symphony orchestras, even though they are much more costly, and less popular, than, say, music festivals. Mill asserted that higher pleasure was more pleasurable, presumably explaining why people would undergo pain (learning) to achieve them. It is hard to find evidence for this. A more plausible idea is that intellectual or moral pleasures are less subject to tolerance or to craving. Going to a fine performance of the opera Wozzeck does not normally lead to an increased desire to hear Berg's music every day of the week. Nor is it followed by initial satiation and then a craving for more. If anything, it is an experience that one can look back on and savour, but perhaps never want to repeat. Eating an ice-cream sundae may have a similar consequence, but is more likely to lead to a desire to repeat the experience, with a guilty feeling that one would like to have four scoops and not just three, and two sauces rather than one.

In *The Subjection of Women* (which, of course, he opposes), Mill (1970: 11) writes about situations in which men understand their wives:

> The woman must be worth knowing, and the man not only a competent judge, but of a character sympathetic in itself, and so well adapted to hers, that he can either read her mind by sympathetic union, or has nothing in himself which makes her shy of disclosing it. Hardly anything can be more rare than this conjunction.

Both Mill and Bentham seem to have had the 'character sympathetic in itself' to which Mill refers in this quotation, and, as I noted previously, Bentham's personal experience was that giving others pleasure gave him pleasure. However, his formulation of utilitarianism did not account for this. Mill thought that other people's pleasure did impact on each of us in three ways. First, he accepted Hume's idea that our upbringing gives us lasting emotional dispositions, so that a well brought-up person, who was told off by their mother for upsetting a playmate, would continue to feel the same pain of being criticized as an adult if they found that they had upset someone. Second, he thought that we often need other people to cooperate with us in achieving our pleasures, and the chances of them doing that are increased if we make sure that they also gain pleasure in the process (this principle has been accepted in social psychology, where it goes under the name of social exchange theory). Neither of these explanations of why we take others into account feels much better than enlightened selfishness.

Mill never quite brought himself to think of sympathy as simply built into us, as Hume did. His detailed consideration in Chapter 3 of *Utilitarianism* (John Stuart Mill, 1867) starts from the premise that we would not have discord in society if sympathy were 'entire', but that many people do not have it. However, those who do have it consider it a 'natural feeling' that is not imposed on them by society or a 'superstition of education' but an attribute, possibly the consequence of social development. Most importantly it is, according to Mill, the 'ultimate sanction of the greatest happiness morality'.

'I feel happy'

The utilitarians were focused on welfare: the happiness of populations, and Aristotle on life satisfaction. Both are more about being rather than feeling happy. I have headed this section with the title of a famous song from the musical *West Side Story* which combines Sondheim's expressive lyrics about happiness and love with music that is infectiously happy. Bernstein's music achieves this by mimicking behaviour we associate with happiness: a quick tempo (young people who are happy often work more quickly), an unusually emphatic beat towards the end of a phrase (an upbeat) that mirrors the emphasis that happy or very confident people put on each word in an utterance, and a lilting dance-like memory that caters for a wish to dance that is often associated with joy.

Feelings of joy that are intense enough to demand our attention are rare. They are exhilarating 'peak experiences' when they come, but they are typically transitory. One can make efforts to prolong them or make them more frequent, but these are usually artificial, and often involve taking drugs, having a lot of sex or doing other risky things. These activities can become ends in themselves as they are often addictive. This means that they require higher 'doses' of the rewarding experience, and that the experience becomes narrower and more idiosyncratic, in which case other people may need to be coerced into participation since the experience is less likely to be rewarding to them. Other people may view the activities as sordid or demeaning and the highs that result promote less and less happiness, however rewarding they remain. Prolonged joy may even become a kind of disease, when it is associated with bipolar disorder.

Maria in *West Side Story*, like her Shakespearean model Juliet, is overwhelmed by her joy and stops thinking about all of the complications of her love for a hated enemy. Feelings obtrude into consciousness when our thoughts are weak or confused. Intense happiness and thoughtlessness often go hand in hand as they do in Maria/Juliet. Joy is often linked to overcoming a deeply felt concern: eating when we are starving, for example, or solving a problem that has been troubling us for some time. Joy narrows our behavioural repertoire so that we focus our attention on resolving the concern. It is motivational. But in this process it may also be, as Sartre described, 'magical'. It reshapes our perception of the world, but sometimes, as Maria/Juliet found, in destructive ways.

Reward

Joy belongs to a cluster of words that includes fun, laughter, gaiety, pleasure, excitement, exhilaration and ecstasy. All of these words would be indications to most people of having a good time, with 'good' meaning 'rewarding' rather than ethically superior. 'Reward' in this context is anything that positively reinforces behaviour: that is, if an animal performs an action that results in, say, being given a food pellet, they are likely to perform the action again, to get another food pellet.

What is pleasing, or rewarding, changes according to the state of our organism. Some things are rewarding because they satisfy a lack, that is an appetite or a desire: when we are thirsty, we are likely to think largely of the pleasure of having a drink. Other things are rewarding because they provide relief from tension, discomfort or pain (Seaford, 2011). On those occasions we may focus on relief. The fact that both can be described as rewards, and that relieving either can be described as making someone feel happy, is confusing, and I will come back to this when I look at 'being happy' in the next chapter.

Rewards, and pleasure, are subject to satiety, unlike happiness. One day of happiness does not reduce the intensity of the next day of happiness, should someone be lucky enough to have two together, any more than one day of sunshine and blue skies reduces the intensity of the sun or the blueness of the sky on a subsequent summer day. But I may take less pleasure from the second day because my appetite for sunshine and blue skies has been diminished. I 'habituate' to my good fortune, to use jargon.

It may be a good thing that we get used even to paradise. Habituation does not occur in the clinical condition of hypomania and untreated hypomania is associated with increased mortality, aggression, relationship breakdown, poor health and injury.

Nor does reward necessarily lead to happiness. We would not suppose that everyone who gets an Olympic Gold medal feels happy, even though all of them receive the same reward. Some winners might be resentful that their race was not properly organized, and that they nearly lost. Others may have just had bad news, which makes their medal seem unimportant. The situation may be even more complicated for winners of the silver medal, who may feel bitter about not winning the gold.

Is happiness just a feeling or a judgement?

We use happy to mean a feeling, and we use it to mean life satisfaction. Unfortunately for our purposes, we can use it to label other people's emotions, too. There is even a signal for it – smiling – so that other people know when we are happy. People being people, it is possible to fake a smile, but this kind of 'social' smiling differs from the involuntary smile associated with happiness. The difference was first noted by the French electrophysiologist Duchenne (Duchenne (de Boulogne), 1876). Social smiles involve the mouth only. A happy smile spreads to the eyes and we can feel that, even if we can't see it. We call it an infectious smile or even, sometimes, a happy smile.

Babies smile from birth. When the author was a baby this was attributed to 'indigestion': to something purely from within, and it is true that the stimulus to these early smiles is unknown. These baby smiles do not necessarily involve the eyes. They are produced fleetingly amidst other similarly fleeting facial expressions, as if these expressions are being practised. However, this kind of smiling quickly changes into responsive smiling, from 2 months old or so. These are 'Duchenne' or true smiles, involving both the eyes and face. Babies smile at this age when their desires are being satisfied, for example after they have been fed, and also when their needs are attended to: after they have been burped or had their nappy changed, for example.

Smiling babies are often called happy babies but, as they get older, different smiles develop that do not indicate happiness. Children learn appeasing smiles, designed to turn away anger or criticism. Girls begin to smile more than boys in adolescence, possibly for this reason (Dodd et al., 1999). This suggests that smiling becomes a less reliable indicator of inner state, and more controlled by social expectation, for which there does appear to be evidence (LaFrance et al., 2003). Smiling is not just culturally but genetically influenced. Children with a more active variant of a gene for a protein that transports a metabolite of serotonin, a transmitter in the brain that is particularly important in the frontal and evolutionarily newer area of the brain, smile more than children with a less active transporter (Grossmann et al., 2011).

So does smiling indicate happiness in adults? Two scientists video-recorded winners of Olympic gold medals when they were on the podium being awarded their medals. They certainly did smile then, but only when they were interacting with someone. Their smiles disappeared when they were just standing there (Fernandez-Dols & Ruiz-Belda, 1995). That might be a consequence of the display rules discussed in the previous paragraph, one of which is that smiling when you are not engaged with someone else is 'fatuous'. It may be that the winners felt a smile welling up inside them, but only allowed it to show when they were interacting, as a kind of thanks to the officials who were rewarding them. So, perhaps, even if displaying a smile might not always be a good indication of happiness, feeling smiley inside might be.

There are inner smiley feelings we might not want to call happy. We might secretly smile because of someone else's misfortune, for example. This kind of feeling, that Nietzsche called by the French term 'ressentiment' but is usually known by the German word, Schadenfreude, has as much anger and contempt about it as it does happy feeling. It is however enough of a positive feeling that people seek it out. We take pleasure in cartoons or stories where someone gets their 'come-uppance', possibly because it is a kind of relief. It is a relief because we might have unpleasant negative feelings like envy or humiliation when we see someone more fortunate than ourselves, and these feelings dissipate if we see that same person in an unenviable or humbling situation.

Smiles are themselves rewarding but, oddly enough, especially if they are fleeting. A brief smile from someone in whom a smile is rare is often more precious than a fixed smile on the face of someone who is perpetually smiling. Not just smiles, but everything connected with pleasure has this same fleeting quality. So much so that Mill wrote in his autobiography, 'Ask yourself whether you are happy, and you cease to be so' (J. S. Mill, 1909: 94).

Feeling joy is what Gilbert Ryle called a 'pang' (Ryle, 2009: 83). It is gone almost as soon as you register it, although because of its intensity the memory of pleasure can often linger. Every aspect of the embodiment of pleasure seems to conduce to this result. Scents are often pleasurable and sometimes give one joy as a result. But nasal mucus contains an enzyme that rapidly oxidizes aldehydes to acids and splits esters to acids and alcohols (Nagashima & Touhara, 2010). Since many floral and fruity scents are either aldehydes or esters, and their corresponding acids and alcohols have much less scent, this means that the perfume of a flower is lost almost as soon as we detect it. We quickly get used to touch, and no longer feel it as pleasurable, although not so quickly to touch in the erogenous areas. Our attention wanders away from the pleasures of eating; and we quickly become tolerant of the pleasurable effects of the most euphoriant drugs, needing to take larger and larger doses to get the same high as we once did. The relief of discomfort can be equally transient.

Is feeling happy any sort of indication of being happy?

It is perhaps for the above reasons that many philosophers have concluded that feeling pleasure is a kind of accident or by-product of living and that, although it may be an indication of whether or not one is living in the right way, to make feeling pleasure as much as possible one's aim is doomed to failure.

Even if genetic engineering made it possible to prevent happiness spontaneously decaying, there are only a few philosophers who would advocate this (one of the advocates is Nick Bostrom who also argues for cybernetic enhancement). Most philosophers would share the intuitions of Robert Nozick. He imagined an 'experience machine' into which we could be hooked, and which would give us continuous pleasure, whilst being unaware of the real world around us (Nozick, 1974). His sense was that few people would actually choose to be in the machine.

Nozick suggests that a world without unhappiness would not be a good world. Other philosophers who take this position often argue that unhappiness is a kind of psychic pain. Pain has survival value. It is essential to our health. People who have no pain receptors in a limb overextend their joints, leading to damage, and wound themselves more severely and with greater risk of neglecting the wound and developing an infection. Negative mental emotions may have a guardian function in our personal and social dealings, comparable to the guard that pain provides to our bodies. Without anxiety or worry, we take too many risks and act without preparation or precaution. Without depression, we over-estimate our energy and capacity, trade too much on other people's esteem for us, and do not learn from our losses to realize what we truly value. George Bernard Shaw voiced the scepticism that many of us have about euphoria, or persistent happiness, when he put this into the mouth of his alter ego, John Tanner, in *Man and Superman*: 'A lifetime of happiness! No man alive could bear it: it would be hell on earth' (from Act 1, scene 2).

This is not to say that we should be careless about unhappiness. Unremitting unhappiness or fear would be as damaging to our health as unremitting happiness. Habituation normally prevents us from feeling persistently unhappy, just as it prevents persistent happiness. But habituation does not always work. Habituation is slower to strong stimuli than to weak, and it can be reversed by other stimuli that lead to the same response as the one that has become habituated (Thompson, 2009). If we apply this to emotion, we might expect that extreme unhappiness does not habituate, and that repeated but different causes of unhappiness prevent habituation.

Neurophilosophy and experimental philosophy

Happiness is, according to many of the philosophers considered in this chapter, tied up not just with pleasure but with life satisfaction, and that is in some way tied up with living well – with the moral approbation of other people. So there is a strong tie-in of happiness and personal morality, and of prescriptions about how to be happy with ethics.

Neurophilosophy (Churchland, 1986) sets out to consider these associations using neuroscience and not speculation. Not everyone is convinced this is wise. Such people argue that the essence of a feeling, its qualia, has, like other aspects of consciousness and indeed psychology, eluded the scanner (Miller, 2010). My discussion of fundamental approaches to happiness ends with the Victorians, not because the discussions have not continued since then, but because most of the main concepts that will figure in this book had been presaged by philosophers by that time. Where philosophers have made subsequent important contributions, I will come back to them in the relevant text.

One of neurophilosophy's most striking paradigms is sometimes formulated as 'the trolley problem', first put forward by Phillipa Foot (Foot, 1967). It tests the extent to which people make utilitarian decisions.

The trolley, and the reverse trolley, problem (there are many variants) is discussed extensively by Peter Singer, who has summarized much of the research, including that by neuroscientists, into the problem in the 20 years since Foot put it forward (Singer, 2005). This is the trolley problem: you are standing on a bridge; you see a trolley rolling down a track that will take it into five people working on the track. It is heavy and will kill at least some of them if you cannot stop it, but there is nothing to stop it with, except the very heavy man standing next to you. Do you throw him over? A variant of the trolley problem, the reverse trolley problem, is that the very heavy man is not standing next to you, but you are standing next to a railway point control switch. The heavy man is still in the problem, but standing across the rails in a siding. You can divert the runaway trolley into the siding with your switch, but doing so will almost certainly kill the heavy man. However, it will spare the five people who are still working on the main track. So, do you divert it?

Pushing the man off the bridge was the preferred option for only 10% of a large sample collected for one study (Bartels & Pizarro, 2011). The reverse trolley solution was much more likely to be chosen. In fact, a majority would have diverted the train into the siding.

In accordance with Mill's idea that one can rely on sympathy to temper the application of the greatest happiness, non-utilitarians who are unwilling to sacrifice the one for the many, are more likely to have compassionate feelings towards other people (Gleichgerrcht & Young, 2013), whilst the utilitarians are more likely to be highly rational, callous, 'Machiavellian' and with a lack of meaning in life. But what is, perhaps, more interesting is not that psychology supports philosophy but that there are links with brain function, suggesting that these reactions are not, as Mill suggested, something we have to think about but something that is wired into our brains, as Harvard academic Joshua Green has advocated in a series of papers. As with all current neuroscience, there are dangers of over-generalizing from the evidence provided by increases or decreases of blood flow in one area or another of the brain, which is what much neuroscience is currently based on (Kahane & Shackel, 2010). There is, though, converging evidence that reduced function in the ventromedial (on the underside and towards the middle) of the prefrontal cortex (the part of the brain above our eyes) is required for the utilitarian judgement inasmuch as people with damage to this part of the brain are more likely to make utilitarian judgements (Moll & de Oliveira-Souza, 2007). It would be wrong though to consider that non-utilitarian judgements are somehow 'higher', as repeated transcranial magnetic stimulation (TMS) to the dorso-lateral prefrontal cortex increases the likelihood of non-utilitarian choices, at least in women (Fumagalli et al., 2010). This part of the brain is also involved in another kind of emotional decision making: paying people back for perceived injustice. In laboratory conditions, in games in which the participants gain financial rewards for cooperative or competitive behaviour, volunteers will pass up some part of their own financial reward in order to reduce the reward of another player who they deem to be unfair. This payback is reduced if the dorso-lateral prefrontal cortex is subject to repeat TMS (Knoch et al., 2008).

The dorso-lateral prefrontal cortex is probably the part of the brain that comes closest to being the substrate of our 'inner voice' or, perhaps even, our 'super-ego'. Of course, these are inappropriate attributions. An inner voice is a subjective experience. The dorso-lateral prefrontal cortex is just a very complicated bit of machinery embedded in a bigger machine. But it seems to need something like 'energy' (probably related to dopaminergic afferents from reward circuits becoming depleted) and when this is at a low level in chronic dieters, they are less likely to control their impulse to eat high-calorie food (Wagner et al., 2013). To my mind, this suggests that the kind of self-control, or at least self-training, promoted by the warrior philosophers presupposes a level of continuous reward that gives them the mental energy to maintain this control. The less powerful may have to make do with only intermittent levels of reward sufficient to maintain self-control and ensure justice and fairness. For them, therefore, immediate reward may be a much greater priority.

2

The Health Economist's Viewpoint

The panic that gripped London during the Great Plague of 1665 is vividly described in Daniel Defoe's *Journal of the Plague Year*. This was not the only plague year, and from 1623 each parish published weekly or monthly figures of deaths in the area that alternately horrified and reassured the parishioners. No one knew what to do, but knowing whether deaths were mounting or falling seemed to give some semblance of control. These bills of mortality continued to be collected in London and elsewhere until they were integrated into national statistics by the creation of a national registry in 1836. The main purpose may have been to formalize marriage records and therefore record lineages, but the first statistician attached to the Registry, William Farr, used the statistics to identify threats to public health, with particular attention paid to cholera, that 19th century plague. The first public health act was passed in 1845 but was repealed. A second, much more effective act that imposed duties on local authorities, was put into law in 1875.

Mortality remains a key indicator of health, but has proven insufficient for 21st century public health. One reason for this is an enormous expansion in the scope of 'health', along with the success of public health itself. As the World Health Organization (WHO) has recognized (Wang, 2012), the burden of disease has shifted from diseases like cholera that either kill you or from which you recover, to diseases and conditions that linger. The public money needed to protect against most infectious diseases is a lot less than the cost of lost production or the cost of the emergency medical care that such diseases lead to. Moreover, infectious diseases spread. Hence, prevention and early intervention, even if costly, are less expensive than the cost of an epidemic. Rationing of health care expenditure is not a significant issue for infectious disease. The same arguments do not hold for chronic disease. Some kind of rationing is inevitable, especially as newer treatments are often much more costly than traditional ones for a small gain in effectiveness.

The medical model, too, has evolved. For a short period, it seemed like one caught something deadly – scarlet fever, perhaps, or TB – then a doctor came along and provided an antibiotic, a specific and usually effective treatment, and one returned to one's former state of health. Even on the crest of the wave of modern medicine that swept the world in the middle of the 20th century, there were reservations. Scarlet fever could, for example, leave the heart valves weakened and result in adult-onset heart disease. But the magic bullets that doctors could deploy against 'germs' did not work on chronic diseases. Sometimes the cure was even worse than the disease, and it was often prohibitively costly. So measures of health were developed that were not just about survival, but about quality of life, and the utilitarians, as it turned out, provided a perfect approach to measuring this.

The psychosocial and bio-psychosocial models of 20th-century psychiatry (Ghaemi, 2009) were a reaction to the infection model of disorder, giving weight to social circumstances, psychological status and biological factors influencing resilience, as well as being attacked by a particular pathogen. Although the bio-psychosocial model was too vague to be generally useful, its general thrust has proven insightful. Mind, body and society are linked. Happiness is a particularly important influence on health and, of course, vice versa.

Although many 19th-century adults were fatalistic about their health, not all were. Some turned to spiritual healing, whilst others turned to exercise, the outdoor life and special diets – much as we do today – to keep pathogens at bay.

Few people ever consider themselves to be completely healthy. We are more tired than we would like to be, or less energetic. The 19th-century exercisers and dieters sometimes discovered that they could feel not just protected by their activities, but healthier than ever before. 'Feeling healthy' emerged as an aim in life to lie alongside 'feeling happy'. Philosophers have not given the same detailed treatment to feeling healthy as they have to feeling happy. No one questions, for example, whether feeling healthy is a spurious goal in the way that feeling happy is called into question. What is notable about the two feelings is that they are often entwined, at least for people who are not actually ill (Mukuria & Brazier, 2013). Not only does chronic ill health increase the risk of unhappiness, but chronic unhappiness increases the risk of poor health, both possibly mediated by the state of the autonomic nervous system (Kok et al., 2013). Many people, too, experience unhappiness in their bodies such that the main symptom of low mood might be a lack of energy, and other people experience depression as the first symptom of the onset of a physical illness.

Utilitarian philosophy has proved of considerable value in dealing with this complexity.

Positive and negative health

When illness strikes, we all seek a remedy for ourselves and even more so for our nearest and dearest but preventing illness and maintaining our and our family's health is a new idea and one that has still not penetrated society. There are people who still believe, as many did in the 19th century, that health is a fate that is handed out, rather than a state that can be cultivated. Use of the word 'health' is sometimes termed a 'negative' one, or a definition by exclusion. Health, on this definition, is the state of not being ill. The newer idea, that health involves more than this, including preventing or minimizing future illness, was captured in a famous definition of health formulated by the World Health Organization when it defined its brief on its foundation in 1946: 'Health is a state of complete physical, mental and social well-being and not merely the absence of disease or infirmity' (WHO, [1946] 2006: 1).

Whether one adopts a positive or negative view of health has implications for behaviour. If one believes that there is a positive state of health that can be maintained by one's own efforts, then prudence about health is justified. If one does not belief this, then one can pray to providence for good health, but there is nothing that one can do about it, until one gets ill. As we saw in Chapter 1, there were comparable contrasting positions about happiness in ancient times, with the Socratics arguing that one should make hay whilst the sun shone, and the Cyrenaics arguing that hay would always turn up during a rainy period, and so the best thing was just to have fun whilst the sun was shining.

The results of a study by the UK Department of Health demonstrate that when it comes to health, opinion is still divided. Structured interviews of nearly 5000 adults were followed by a series of focus groups and qualitative interviews (Department of Health, 2010a). The results are summarized in Figure 2.1.

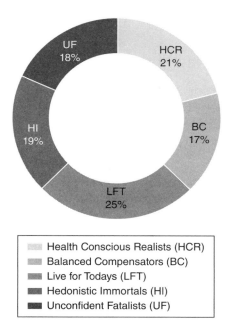

Figure 2.1 Segmenting the population by categories of health-related attitudes and behaviour

Source: Department of Health, 2010a, *Healthy foundations life-stage segmentation model toolkit.* London: Department of Health.

There are substantial economic, social and psychological differences between the groups, as summarized in Figure 2.2.

	Health Conscious Realists	Balanced Compensators	Live for Todays	Hedonistic Immortals	Unconfident Fatalists
Value health	High	High	Med	Low	Med
Control over health	High	High	Med	Med	Low
Healthy lifestyle is easy/enjoyable	High	High	Low	Med	Low
Health fatalism	Low	Med	High	Low	High
Risk taking	Low	High	Med	High	Med
Short termism	Low	Med	High	Low	High
Self esteem	High	High	Med	High	Low

Key:

More positive motivation

More negative motivation

Figure 2.2 Summary of motivational differences between the motivation segments

Source: Department of Health, 2010a, *Healthy foundations life-stage segmentation model toolkit.* London: Department of Health.

Most of us would seek to remedy a persisting state of unhappiness, much as we would seek a cure for illness. But most of us would also try to increase our happiness, and that would include preventing or minimizing future unhappiness, in all the ways that I discussed in Chapter 1. The notion that there is something called health that is not just being without illness, but includes preventing or minimizing future illness and is partly under our control, is much more recent than this idea of happiness. I would go so far as to say that attitudes towards health have lagged behind attitudes towards happiness for millennia, and, as the Department of Health research shows, many people still think that ill health is just something that happens, a misfortune. Philosophers did not begin to focus on health as a goal or aim of living until the 19th century, and then it was the duty of governments to take account of the health of the citizenry. It took the advent of modern medicine, principally antibiotics, to give people the sense that illness and therefore health can be controlled. Health, like happiness, is consequently recast as a property and not as a gift.

Utilities

In their founding definition, the World Health Organization ([1946] 2006) was reflecting another shift in thinking: that health and well-being are intimately linked. Bentham anticipated this by basing his ethical philosophy on the avoidance of pain and seeking of pleasure, conceived as one dimension of felicific calculus: a philosophy on pleasure and pain that could encompass both mental and physical pain, and the pleasure of bodily experience, as well as the pleasures of reading, listening to music, doing good, and so on.

Bentham's felicific calculus (1876) works well because it makes no distinction between the pain of mental suffering and that of physical suffering, or between the pleasures of playing Beethoven sonatas and of eating chocolate ice cream. Pleasure so defined can encompass both feeling healthy and feeling happy. Not everyone is seeking pleasure or avoiding suffering all of the time, but only a very small number of people would prefer pain to pleasure as a general rule and of those, we might say that they take pleasure in pain. Pain can be generalized to include any aversive state, and pleasure to include any reward, yet both can still be quantified or at least ranked by asking a person or many people to say which is worse and which is better. Individual ranks may differ from each other but for a large sample – such as a population for whose health a public health professional is responsible – a stable average ranking can be calculated (Daniel Kahneman, 2006), for example by asking the people surveyed which outcomes are preferred.

There are several methods of obtaining rankings or, as they are termed by health economists, utilities. One, the 'standard gamble' method, involves writing a vignette of a particular state of health, giving clear indications of the different symptoms and restrictions to normal living associated with it, and then asking a person to gamble on being in this state versus being dead or being completely healthy. Bennett et al. (2000), for example, devised descriptions of four states of depression. In the most severe, the affected person (wording taken from the paper, but with slight modifications):

1. Feels terribly down or sad all the time; doesn't enjoy anything and feels desperate.
2. Feels worthless and sees absolutely no hope, and/or doesn't know why people even care, and/or feels very guilty about the past and sees no future.
3. Feels like their mind is shut down, overloaded or racing; can't read or watch TV and can't make even little decisions.
4. Has terrible sleep these days and doesn't feel rested; has absolutely no energy and feels constantly tired; has no interest in food, and has lost a lot of weight over the past month (more than 5% of body weight).
5. Can't do anything; is completely shut down, and/or extremely agitated, and/or thinking of suicide constantly and having thoughts or making plans to end life.
6. Has had to stop work and/or do nothing at home, and/or completely withdraw. (2000: 1172)

Bennett et al. asked a group of people who were recovering from depression to compare being in a state of severe depression to being perfectly healthy, or to being dead. The comparison was made quantitative using a technique derived from game theory (Von Neumann & Morgenstern, 1953). Each participant was asked: 'If you could enter a lottery, and have 9 chances out of 10 of winning perfect health for the rest of your life, but 1 chance in 10 of dying, would you do it?' If the person says 'yes', they are then asked: 'If you could either take a gamble on the lottery or be severely depressed for the rest of your life, which would you choose?' The questions are asked repeatedly with varying probabilities, until the person is just as willing to take the lottery as to have lifelong severe depression. The assumption is that a person who is offered the choice of perfect health and the lottery would go for the lottery if the probability of death was nil and the probability of perfect health was 1. So the utility of perfect health (utilities are weights, so they are always expressed as a number between 0 and 1) is 1. If death is being compared to the lottery, then any probability, however faint, of perfect health offered by the lottery would be better. So the utility of death is 0. Bennett et al. (2000) found that the utility, averaged across their sample, of severe, lifelong depression was little higher than death: 0.04.

This result accords with our idea of depression that it is not just an absence of pleasure (that would be anhedonia), but a presence of constant psychic pain, made worse by participation in any activity that puts one in touch with this pain – and that is almost every activity that causes any kind of self-reflection. Feeling that any aspect of living brings pain understandably makes death an attractive option.

Studies to determine utilities are time-consuming. However, this effort can be reduced if it is assumed that different samples of the population will each arrive at the same utility estimate. (As noted previously, this assumption works best when individual decisions are not being considered, but how a group of people will choose.) If this is assumed, then a questionnaire can be used that has been previously weighted so that the score can be 'converted' into utilities. The method is similar to that adopted by Bennett et al., but rather than focusing on depression it focuses on a wide range of symptoms and activities. An example is the 12-item reduced version (SF-6D) of the Nottingham health questionnaire (SF-36).

Even though the results of the Bennett et al. (2000) study accord with our intuitions, the standard gamble method obviously requires a good deal of thought by the participants, and 1 in 10 people in the study had to be excluded because they did not understand it. There are other, simpler, methods for estimating utilities, but none of them are free of another, more fundamental objection: we are none of us the rational choosers that Von Neumann and Morgenstern imagine. In real life, we may make different choices to those that we say we would make in the abstract, and, if we are healthy, we value our health less than if we are ill.

Kahneman and Tversky studied economic decision making when there is limited information about the likely outcomes of decisions, and formulated an influential prospect theory (Tversky & Kahneman, 1974). This accounts better for the everyday basis of decision making than does a fully rational theory. Tversky and Kahneman noted, for example, that changes in fortune (gains or losses) influence decisions more than the final amount the person has, as a result of their decision. Small probabilities also tend to be amplified and large probabilities reduced, and losses have more impact on decision making than gains of the same amount (Daniel Kahneman & Tversky, 1979).

The bottom line, according to Kahneman, is that people cannot be relied on to make the choices that will be most to their advantage. He advocates a return to 'experience utilities': looking not at what people choose, but what will bring the most pleasure with the least pain; in short, a return to Bentham's (1876) utility theory. This suggestion has been rejected by many economists.

Health, quality of life and utility

Allowing people to choose between health states enables many more factors to be included in those health states than just symptoms. People can be asked, for example, whether they would prefer to be mildly depressed or to experience the side-effects of antidepressants, which often include some degree of blunting of feeling.

Health care up until the 1970s focused on saving lives. The main outcome of health care was whether one lived or died, and being healthy was a matter of living one's normal allotted span. But health care, and health prevention, became so good at saving lives that chronic conditions – those that produce pain or disability but not death – became increasingly important. Health care began to be judged not just on whether it saved lives, but also on the quality of lives it saved. The problem was how to weight some pain with lots of disability versus moderate pain and low disability, to take just one example. Utilities provide the answer so long as it is accepted that pain from any source and pleasure from any source can be weighed up in the same way. Bentham thought so – but of course Aristotle did not.

Rating scales

It is not necessary to judge the utility of any particular health state *de novo*. As noted above, once weights have been attached to rating scales, it is assumed that the answers to the scale can be converted to utilities. So the utility of any particular health state, for the population as a whole, can be estimated by having a large enough sample of people complete the appropriate rating scale. This indirect method tends to obscure one of the larger assumptions made in the estimating utilities: that utilities are estimated with reference to points. These are usually death at one end of the scale, and perfect health at the other. Death is a very clear reference point for many people (although few of us can imagine what our own death will be like), but perfect health presents difficulties if Aristotle is right (as we think that he is) and perfect health is context bound and not absolute.

What use are utilities?

Quality of life estimates have had an incalculable impact on health services, because they enable the value of health interventions to be expressed monetarily. This is often achieved by estimating a quality adjusted life year (QALY). Suppose we consider a year spent in a health state with a utility of 0.5. We could think of this as equivalent to half of the days of the year spent as, effectively, dead and half of the year spent in perfect health. In other words, being in a health state with a utility of 0.5 is like each year being as healthy as half a year of someone with perfect health. Going back to our severe depression example, where the utility is 0.04, a person in that state can expect a reduction of 96% in their quality of life years. If they have 48 years of actual life left, this means that they have the equivalent of only six months of full quality, or a reduction of 47.5 quality life years. Suppose though that antidepressant treatment, which takes three months to be fully effective, improves the person's health state to a utility of 0.8 (remembering that drugs are never completely effective and always have some side-effects, so a return to perfect health cannot be expected). The person who takes antidepressants can now expect 0.25 x 0.04 plus 47.75 x 0.8 QALYs or just over 37.8 QALYs, a gain of over 37 QALYs. There are various ways of estimating the monetary value of a QALY. The UK agency, the National Institute of Clinical and Health Excellence, operates on a value of between £20,000 and £30,000 per QALY. This is probably derived from the loss of income plus the cost of government benefits of someone not working for a year.

QALYs enable the rational use of resources. For example, the cost of treating severe depression can be calculated for each QALY gained, and compared with the cost per QALY gained for treating moderate depression. The comparison (Simon et al., 2006) is very much in favour of treating severe depression (cost per QALY gained is £5777 at 2002–3 prices) rather than moderate depression (cost per QALY is £14,540), indicating that – if there has to be a choice – the most efficient use of health resources in depression would be to focus on the early detection and treatment of severe depression.

Well-being and social capital

The utility approach can be applied, economists have argued, to happiness as well as to health. Moreover, it can be used to combine health and happiness in a well-being index. The rationale for doing this is set out in various national well-being initiatives. The first such initiative was in 1972 by Bhutan, and its King, Jigme Singye Wangchuck, who commissioned a Gross Happiness Index as a preferable measure of Bhutan's development to the usual calculation of gross output, the gross domestic product (GDP). An index has been developed that is consistent with traditional Buddhist values, including, for example, the impact of development on the environment and on social life. It has attracted the interest of many other countries, and the then prime minister of Bhutan, Jigmi Y Thinley, was invited to address the UN General Assembly in 2011 about the index.

Following Bhutan's example, there have been surveys of well-being in many countries (although Bhutan's focus on well-being has been dropped since the People's Democratic Party came to power there in the summer of 2013).

The French 'Commission on the Measurement of Economic Performance and Social Progress' was created by the then President of France, Nicolas Sarkozy, in 2008. Its work was directed by two academics from US universities, Joseph Stiglitz and Amartya Sen, and a French academic, Jean Fitoussi. Its main conclusions (Stiglitz et al., 2009) were that there was a growing distrust of the Gross Domestic Product as a measure of national wealth, because it did not tally with the individual's perception of how well off they were themselves. Like Bhutan, the commission thought that this had to do with the sustainability of economic development (although they offered little evidence that most individuals worried about this), but also because increased production did not lead to increased well-being.

Governments are there to organize collective institutions and initiate collective actions. Sociologists argue about whether governments act for all the people, all the people who elect them or for a minority who reward them with patronage or are simply the class from which the government is drawn. An alternative model to this one of government self-interest is enshrined in the codes of human rights that have been developed by the United Nations and in Europe by the Council of Europe and, most recently, by the European parliament. These codes formulate a government's parental responsibilities to its citizens, an idea first put forward by Thomas Jefferson (Jefferson, 1903), who considered that 'the care of human life and happiness ... is the only legitimate objective of good government' (ibid., p. 359, but speech actually delivered in 1809). The Sarkozy commission took for granted that these parental responsibilities included not just health but also the well-being of its citizenry.

The economic argument put forward for this concern is based on a simple parenting value: parents want to leave their children better off than they were. Better off in this instance includes not just liquidity – money – but better stock – capital – from which money can be made in the future. Capital in this instance includes more trees and more productive farmland, in other words a better 'environment' (hence the emphasis on sustainability). It also includes the social environment. Insecurity is one particular aspect of this.

Capital for well-being also includes workers who are able to undertake the more complex tasks required of them by development and who will work with fewer days off, show more initiative and not waste energy in conflict. The workforce needs therefore to be happy, as well as healthy, but also well educated. Increasing the well-being of the workforce should, the commission argued, be high on any government's agenda because a productive workforce can be seen, pace Marx, as a kind of capital.

The mental wealth of nations

This notion that citizens are a kind of wealth belonging to the government, directly informed another government project, this time in the UK. The idea of the Foresight project was to put together the science available in 2007 to set priorities for research and investment in key areas linked to future welfare or wealth. One of these was called the Foresight project on mental capital and well-being. A report, published in *Nature* (Beddington et al., 2008), was entitled 'The mental wealth of nations'. The distinguished authors concluded that mental wealth was composed of mental capital or 'brain power' and mental well-being. Brain power included learning ability, as well as amount of learning, but also something called 'emotional intelligence', social skill and resilience. Some of what the authors called 'key findings' (although they were not findings so much as guesses about what might be worthwhile priorities) are summarized in Figure 2.3.

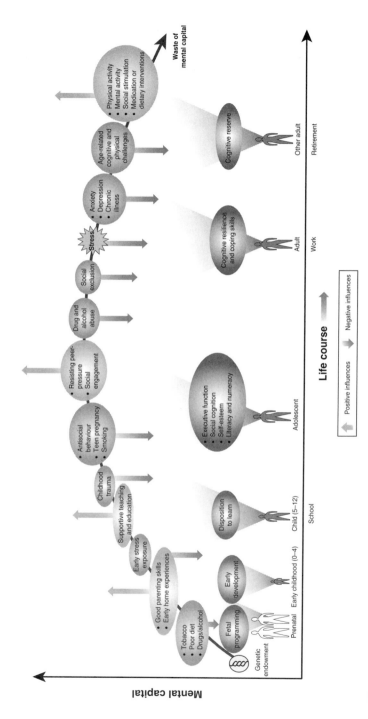

Figure 2.3 Mental capital over the course of life

Source: Beddington et al., 2008, The mental wealth of nations. *Nature,* 455(7216), 1057–1060.

Social capital

A well-informed government would not stop at mental wealth. Research suggests that the well-being of those people who live close to a person influences their well-being. So a further kind of capital that a caring and farsighted government should consider, and which several have, is this kind of 'social capital'. Work on measuring social capital has been carried out by the World Bank and by the UN Office for Economic Development and Capital. The OECD definition of social capital, adopted by the Office for National Statistics in the UK, is 'networks together with shared norms, values and understandings that facilitate co-operation within or among groups' (Keeley, 2007: 103).

Trying to measure everything

Social capital, environmental security, education, individual well-being: can all of these be measured? The OECD thinks so, and has even produced an index – the Better Life Index. However, even with this compendium, aspects of well-being are missed. The most recent version considers inequality: the differences in well-being within a country between the lowest and highest scorers on the index. This is important because, as it turns out, keeping up with the Joneses is one of the scourges of a settled society, and never more so than now when the lifestyle of the Joneses is being presented to us in so many in-your-face ways (we are thinking of television, radio, newspapers, but also Facebook, Twitter, the blogosphere, Flickr, etc.).

Measuring the scope of well-being

Economists, like those in the Sarkozy commission, assume that well-being is a measurable amount, although accepting that only some of it is 'liquid', i.e. having an effect in the present. Utilities do not help in determining which elements of life provide well-being. For example, curvy buildings make people feel better than rectilinear ones (Vartanian et al., 2013) but few measures of well-being include the curviness of one's home or office in their data collection. They tend, in fact, to focus on a rather traditional set of factors such as health, employment, education, income and security (Dolan et al., 2011). Many of these objective measures are included in declarations of human rights, too. Although there are many studies that demonstrate that each of these factors is associated with both happiness and health, there is no empirical study, so far as I know, to work out a top ten of the well-being components. Nowadays, this is likely to include broadband access; access to fresh water seems important worldwide, too, as does a low level of corruption.

Measuring the amount of well-being

Utilities are expensive to calculate, and economists have sometimes used proxy preference measures, for example assuming that as money enables people to purchase their preferred goods, that income could therefore be used as a proxy measure. As we have seen, however, absolute income does not correlate very strongly with well-being.

'Subjective', i.e. self-rated, well-being may be used alongside objective measures or may be used on its own. Subjective measures are increasingly used in national comparisons, as well as in studies of individuals. Some of the most extensive research on subjective well-being has been undertaken by Ed Diener and his co-workers. Diener and Emmons consider that subjective well-being has three separable components: good feelings, bad feelings (they do not assume, unlike Bentham that good and bad are unidimensional) and evaluations of one's life: 'life satisfaction' (Diener & Emmons, 1984). Life satisfaction may be more closely linked to family life, and positive feelings to income, at least for men (Selezneva, 2011).

The Easterlin paradox

Mr Micawber's recipe for happiness was that his annual income should be twenty pounds, but his annual expenditure six pence less. Dickens was advancing a more complex model of happiness than Bentham's. Even if we consider that the want of money is a kind of pain, Dickens' model was not of a continuous spectrum between pain and pleasure but a step function. Once a want is satisfied, it drops out of the equation. Wants satisfied twice over do not make a person any happier than those wants being satisfied by just enough. Mr Micawber was a sanguine, happily married man with a high degree of sociability and bonhomie. He is perhaps not the best person on which to base a theory of happiness as his natural state was happiness, and it was only the want of money that depressed him. Even without being in want, many people may still be unhappy. But repeated cross-sectional comparisons of countries, and analyses of time-series data for specified countries, are consistent with the Micawber principal: increases or decreases in GDP have a short-term effect on national happiness but, except for the least developed countries (Helliwell & Barrington-Leigh, 2010), there may be much less long-term correlation (although there is considerable disagreement about how much) between an increase in a country's income over time and an increase in that country's happiness. Higher GDP is to some degree compensated for by the rising prices of goods, but not wholly. So an increase in buying power and an accumulation of possessions may not mean more happiness once one is over the threshold of want (Easterlin et al., 2010). But, having said that, there is a continuing tendency throughout the world for economic migration: for people to migrate from countries with low GDP to countries with higher GDP. Perhaps they are not seeking happiness for themselves, but for their children. Not everyone agrees with what is called the 'Easterlin paradox': that richer people are happier than poorer people, but that as richer people get even richer, if their country is booming, they do not get even happier.

One reason that Easterlin's observations may not fully apply is that increased average income does not necessarily abolish want. This will also depend on the distribution of wealth. The Easterlin paradox does not mean that income is unimportant. Better-paid people rate their well-being more highly than lower-paid people in every country. But well-being may be linked to relative position: whether or not a person is keeping up with the Joneses. An increase in national prosperity tends to increase everyone's income (although the recent trend in Europe is that the higher paid are now even better paid than their lower-income neighbours). So an increase in national prosperity does not increase relative income, and therefore has no or only a small (economists differ) effect on well-being (I return to this in Chapter 5, on the politician's viewpoint).

Is well-being quantifiable?

Correlations or regressions are the basic methods of analysis that produce the data cited in the previous paragraph. They are based on very large samples and are presented with a high degree of scientific precision, but they are numbers. One number is an estimate of the monetary value of a country's production in a year (GDP). The other is a number based on various estimates of a quantity of happiness, well-being or life satisfaction. Although money is a symbol, it is a very accurate one. I can buy twice as many things with two pounds as I can buy with one. Bentham argued that happiness is 'scalar' in the same way. Dickens' Mr Micawber did not think so: the 6d that distinguishes an income of £19, 19 shillings and sixpence from outgoings of 20 shillings, is a much larger amount than that between an income of £20 and sixpence and the same outgoings. I agree with Mr Micawber. But can a number provide us with a useful approximation, at least at a population level?

To answer this, we need to consider in more detail what economists are measuring. The UK government instructed the Office for National Statistics to survey happiness in the UK (health has been measured since the 19th century, as I noted earlier). Four measures were chosen after expert advice was taken followed by a public consultation: 'Overall, how satisfied are you with your life nowadays?'; 'Overall, to what extent do you feel the things you do in your life are worthwhile?'; 'Overall, how happy did you feel yesterday?'; and 'Overall, how anxious did you feel yesterday?'.

The results of the national survey using these questions were reported in 2012 and continue to be reported regularly on the web pages of the UK Office for National Statistics. (The survey is still continuing, but as part of a bigger survey about employment.) Correlations with predicted data did suggest that the questions had some validity. For example, there was the expected association with intimate relationships (adults who are married, in a civil partnership or cohabiting report higher average ratings of life satisfaction, happiness yesterday and worthwhile life than those who are single, widowed, divorced, separated or formerly in a civil partnership, but there were exceptions); living with children increased self-ratings of how worthwhile life was; and people who were long-term unemployed had lower ratings for life satisfaction, happiness yesterday and life being worthwhile. Life satisfaction was lower for people living in London, and for those who described themselves as Black British, Caribbean or African.

Most of us would conclude that the survey has some face validity, given these associations, although the direction of the correlations, and the possible presence of hidden factors that really account for the associations, remains unknown. But it would be ill-advised for an individual to take them as a prescription for action. Divorcing a violent partner may increase individual well-being, as may moving to London to take up a better job there.

Public health

Public health began with sanitation and the prevention of epidemic infectious disease. It moved on to factory conditions (prevention of accidents), air and water quality, vaccination policies and the legal powers to detain known vectors of infectious diseases. Mental health was first recognized as a public health issue in the UK in the 1930s by the appointment of the psychiatrist Mapperly to the post of consultant psychiatrist and public health physician in Nottingham. Public health has taken some time to shift away from a concern with infectious or acute disease towards chronic disease, but, as it has done so, it has had to take much more account of social factors such as quality of housing, social class, stigma and income inequality which influence the impact of chronic disease. Quality of life and the use of utilities have, as a result, become much more important measures to many public health physicians than life expectancy (although the two can be combined by calculating the expectancy of quality of life years or disability-free years). (I will look in more detail at how public health teams apply these concepts in Chapter 4.)

Choices and happiness

The UK government commissioned the ONS survey because they wanted guidance on how to carry out their role as parents of the country; or perhaps because they wanted to increase well-being and so be re-elected; or because they wanted to move the UK up the league tables. Whatever the reason, the intention was to use the data to take some informed action. One of the prime movers in this was the academic economist and government lobbyist, Lord Richard Layard. He is a follower of Bentham both theoretically and in terms of Bentham's zeal to change things for the better. His ideas about the impact of economics on the public good are contained in a book (P. R. G. Layard, 2011), but are anticipated in a series of Lionel Robbins memorial lectures that he gave in 2003 at the London School of Economics. He concluded that taxes should be high enough to disincentivize working long hours, that government should foster leisure, that job security is more important than pruning the occupants of positions who are not thought to be producing and, most importantly, that spending on mental health should increase substantially. As a result of this, spending has been increased on talking treatments, to target the anxiety and depressive disorders that Layard identified as being priority areas because of their substantial effect on personal and national well-being. Spending on mental health in the UK still lags behind other areas of health spending, however.

Conclusions

Health economists have imagined means of measurement of previously imponderable, but highly valued, qualities of life. By doing so, they have brought happiness, health and well-being into the public arena, making them the concerns of governments as well as individuals and families, and giving public health physicians the tools to deal with the chronic illnesses that have become the main illness burden in the developed world. I have simplified a very large and dynamic field in this chapter, and sometimes minimized the disputes over the conclusions that can be drawn from economics. But there is enough consensus amongst economists to ensure that they now influence government policy all over the world. If there is one single conclusion that has had the biggest effect, it is the paradoxical one that money is not the answer to health or happiness. Spending more does not always ensure greater health in the population, and earning more does not very often produce greater happiness.

Health economists start out with the assumption that perfect health and perfect happiness are measurable states. It seems to me that they are more like limits to which we aspire and, like many limits, as we approach good health or great happiness, our aspirations for health and happiness may change to something else.

One reason for this is that we think of ourselves differently. Our values change. Lord Layard (2011) considers values in the last of his three Robbins memorial lectures, quoting with approval the advice that Jeremy Bentham gave to the daughter of a friend: 'Create all the happiness you are able to create: remove all the misery you are able to remove. Every day will allow you to add something to the pleasure of others, or to diminish something of their pains. And for every grain of enjoyment you sow in the bosom of another, you shall find a harvest in your own bosom; while every sorrow which you pluck out from the thoughts and feelings of a fellow creature shall be replaced by beautiful peace and joy in the sanctuary of your soul' (quoted by Layard, ibid.).

Layard (2011) thinks that this is 'pretty good advice' because a happy society is one in which people have an instinct for right actions, and that is provided by morality. Layard further believes, like Comte, that morality should be founded on altruism. I will consider objections to altruism in Chapter 7. The point though is that Layard (2011) does not consider that economists can tell us how to live, but only tell us what some of the consequences are of how we have chosen to live.

Economics cannot therefore do any better than philosophy at telling us how we can choose a happier or healthier life. Perhaps experts on emotions and health can do better. We will see how they do in the next two chapters, on the psychologist's and doctor's viewpoints.

3

The Psychologist's Viewpoint:
How Happy Are You?

'I feel happy'

This famous song from the musical *West Side Story* combines Sondheim's expressive lyrics about happiness and love with music that is infectiously happy. Bernstein's music achieves this by mimicking behaviour we associate with happiness: a quick tempo (young people who are happy often work more quickly), an unusually emphatic beat towards the end of a phrase (an upbeat) that mirrors the emphasis that happy or very confident people put on each word in an utterance, and a lilting dance-like memory that caters for the wish to dance that is often associated with joy.

In our experience, and in that of other people to whom we have spoken, the feeling of joy (for the moment, let's assume that joy and happiness are much the same) is characteristic and easily recognizable. Perhaps that would be a more reliable indication of happiness? However, the same problems arise as with smiling. People might dance a jig on the fresh grave of a hated enemy, or at least they may look forward to doing so. People might also feel joyful when they see pictures of harm coming to people they hate, or take pleasure in going out of their way to spread damaging rumours about someone they dislike.

Feelings of joy that are intense enough to demand our attention are rare. They are exhilarating 'peak experiences' when they come, but they are typically transitory. One can make efforts to prolong them or make them more frequent, but they are usually artificial, and often involve taking drugs, having a lot of sex or doing other risky things. These activities can become ends in themselves as they are often addictive. This means that they require higher 'doses' of the rewarding experience, and that the experience becomes narrower and more idiosyncratic, in which case other people may need to be coerced into participation since the experience is less likely to be rewarding to them. Other people may view the activities as sordid or demeaning and the highs that result become less and less happy, however rewarding they remain.

Prolonged joy may even become a kind of disease, when it is associated with bipolar disorder, for example.

Maria in *West Side Story*, like her Shakespearean model Juliet, is overwhelmed by her joy and stops thinking about all of the complications of her love for a hated enemy. Feelings obtrude into consciousness when our thoughts are weak or confused. Intense happiness and thoughtlessness often go hand in hand as they do for Maria/Juliet. Joy is often linked to overcoming a deeply felt concern: eating when we are starving, for example, or solving a problem that has been troubling us for some time. Joy narrows our behavioural repertoire so that we focus our attention on resolving the concern. It is motivational. But in this process it may also be, as Sartre described, 'magical'. It reshapes our perception of the world, sometimes, as Maria/Juliet found, in destructive ways.

Reward

Joy belongs to a cluster of words that includes fun, laughter, gaiety, pleasure, excitement, exhilaration and ecstasy. All of these words would be indications to most people of having a good time, with 'good' meaning 'rewarding' rather than ethically superior. 'Reward' in this context is anything that positively reinforces behaviour: that is, if an animal performs an action that results in, say, being given a food pellet, they are likely to perform the action again, to get another food pellet.

What is pleasing, or rewarding, changes according to the state of our organism. Some things are rewarding because they satisfy a lack, that is an appetite or a desire: when we are thirsty, we are likely to think largely of the pleasure of having a drink. Other things are rewarding because they provide relief from tension, discomfort or pain. On those occasions we may focus on relief. The fact that both can be described as rewards, and that relieving either can be described as making someone feel happy, is, we think, confusing, and we come back to this when we look at 'being happy' in the next chapter.

Jane is happy-go-lucky. People find her fun. She does well in her job because of her infectious gaiety and ability to get on with everyone. There is no shortage of money and she can afford to rent a really nice apartment. She likes a good night out and has been known to pass out with drink afterwards. There is always a good-looking man after Jane, and although she is usually up for a fling, she makes sure that she has no long-term entanglements. Jane would say that she is lucky because she enjoys almost everything about her life. If you ask Jane how often she wakes up happy, she would say, 'Almost every day'. If you ask her if she is healthy, she would say that she must be because she hardly ever has a day off sick and only has to go to the doctor a few times a year.

Jane is lucky enough to have a very fond mother who told Jane, when she first left home to go off to university, 'Be happy, dear'.

Most of us would think that Jane is a happy being. She obviously has a greater tendency to feel happy than unhappy. The ratio of the two is sometimes called the hedonic balance and her balance is obviously positive. But has she carried out her mother's injunction to 'be' happy? I am not going to reprise the arguments in Chapter 1 about Jane seeming to discount long-term gratification for immediate reward. It is not clear at this stage of her life whether her enjoyment of having fun and partying will have stood in the way of her acquiring the foundations of longer-term happiness.

There is strong evidence that inborn, temperamental factors are correlated with hedonic balance. One widely accepted way of classifying temperament is into five independent dimensions – the so-called Big Five: openness to experience, consci-entiousness, extraversion, agreeableness and neuroticism (or proneness to anxiety). Our scores on these dimensions do not vary much through life, and they influence us in many different ways. High scores on neuroticism are linked to a pessimistic outlook which, understandably, pushes our hedonic balance into the negative; cheer-fulness, linked to extraversion, pushes it the other way (Schimmack et al., 2004). Measures that are widely accepted by the scientific community (we will come back to what these are) have been given repeatedly to large groups and the scores are shown to vary between individuals but to remain stable over time for each individual (with a significant minority of exceptions) (Fujita & Diener, 2005). Measures given to iden-tical twins also show substantial correlation or 'concordance' (Lykken & Tellegen, 1996). Another way of putting this is that each of us has a hedonic balance set-point that is genetically determined, meaning that some of us are cheerful and that oth-ers of us are gloomy most of the time. We may be pushed off balance by a fortunate or unfortunate event, but over a short period of time we will mostly return to our previous balance point. There are some analogies with health. An acute illness will make us unhealthy but we generally overcome it and return to our previous state of health, whatever that was, although there are some illnesses that cause lasting dam-age. Similarly, there are some life events that may also result in lasting damage or loss that shifts hedonic balance to a gloomier set-point. Marital breakdown (Lucas et al., 2003) and persistent disability (Lucas, 2007) may have this effect. The evidence that good fortune shifts hedonic balance towards happiness is less strong. Couples who feel happier for months before and after the birth of a baby have drifted back to their previous hedonic level by the time their child is 2 years old (Dyrdal & Lucas, 2013).

The genetic model of the hedonic balance is opposed to Bentham's (1876) more commonsense idea, that happiness is just the sum of positive/happy and negative/ unhappy feelings, and that these are linked to our circumstances. One way of recon-ciling Bentham's situational model with the genetic one is to assume that feelings of happiness or unhappiness that are reactions to circumstances do not last. The memory of happiness or unhappiness normally fades with time, but more importantly we get used – habituate – to being happy or unhappy under normal circumstances (we consider abnor-mal circumstances below). Once the acute feelings have faded, we return to our ordinary range of feelings in response to everyday events, a range that is determined by our hereditary temperament. Habituation is the reason that some psychologists consider that we are on a 'hedonic treadmill' (Brickman & Campbell, 1971), but, as we have just seen, we only have to run to regain our peak happiness; if we dawdle instead but we are naturally cheerful and optimistic, we will still be pretty happy.

A re-analysis of national surveys conducted in Germany, Japan, Switzerland and the UK confirms the habituation effect but also suggests that there is a third factor (Bottan & Perez Truglia, 2011). This third factor is the effect that experience has on our disposition towards happiness and therefore on our hedonic balance. Past happiness may create a lasting tendency to feel happy in the future, and past unhappiness may create a lasting gloom.

Our ordinary experience is that although we meet people who make light of disaster, we also meet people who seem crushed by it. Some of them were cheerful and optimistic before the disaster happened. We also meet people who are ground down by being in the wrong job, or in the wrong relationship, or who, without any obvious reason, become profoundly and irremediably depressed. Happiness cannot all be genetically determined.

How important is being happy?

Steptoe and Wardle (2011) asked 5915 participants in the English Longitudinal Study of Aging to complete a logbook of their mood over one day. They were asked to rate, from 1 to 4, how happy, excited or content they were (positive emotions) and how worried, anxious or fearful they were (negative emotions) and 3953 did so. They were asked to do this when they woke, half an hour after they woke, at 7pm and at bedtime, and the ratings at each of these time periods were combined to provide a snapshot of mood experienced over a day. Women were slightly less likely to be in the highest positive affect group; married people were more likely to be in the highest positive affect group; and there were negative correlations with depression and self-rated poor health. Notably, 7.3% of the lowest positive affect group died during the follow-up period (five years on average) compared to a mortality of 3.6% in the highest positive affect group. The difference was less but still significant when the influence of factors that were correlated with both higher mortality and low positive affect was removed. Depression, but not negative feelings, was also correlated with higher mortality.

Happiness and health

Many other studies have shown that the frequency of positive emotions is associated with life expectancy (Diener & Chan, 2011). The frequency of negative feelings is not linked to health, so long as those feelings do not develop into depression. These findings are widely interpreted to mean that happiness increases health; it might also mean that health is a pre-condition for happiness, although longitudinal studies do not support this interpretation (Proulx & Snyder-Rivas, 2013). Another possibility is that a third factor might cause them both. Income is the factor that has been most often canvassed although it does not fit the bill too well for those living above the poverty line (as we discussed in the last chapter), but environment may also cause negative affect as well as ill health. Environmental factors may be physical, such as not having enough food or water, or being cold and damp at home; psychological, such as living with the threat of violence or persistent conflict; habits, such as exercise or alcohol use; or psychosocial, including social inequality (Department of Health, 2010b).

There are many interactions between these components. For example, substantial levels of negative feelings may result in depression, and this reduces life satisfaction, self-rated health and life expectancy (Mykletun et al., 2009). There are also interactions with other factors that may determine well-being, for example those that economists consider to be objective indicators of well-being, such as employment security, family stability, and so on (a fuller list was given in Chapter 2).

Well-being and psychology

'Representative population surveys have repeatedly found that 90% of people report themselves as either "happy" or "very happy" (Myers, 2000) although psychology could say most about the 10% of people for whom this statement was not true' (Wood and Tarrier, 2010: 829). This is how two clinical psychologists describe a 'vacuum' in psychology research and practice in the second half of the last century. There were individual practitioners, especially within the humanistic or existential tradition, who were formulating psychological theories of the good life, but they attracted little of the research funding that clinical psychologists, researching psychological disorders, are able to attract. Perhaps vacua press to be filled, or perhaps the new century brought less willingness to think about the negatives and more willingness to focus greedily on the positives. For whatever reason, the situation has changed now, with the growth of what is often called the positive psychology movement.

Positive psychology

The positive psychology movement was explicitly launched by the psychologist Martin Seligman when chair of the American Psychological Association at the end of the last century, and funded by a large but at the time anonymous grant from Atlantic Philanthropies. Seligman originally focused on what makes for 'authentic happiness' (M. E. P. Seligman, 2003). He has moved on since, and now thinks (M. E. P. Seligman, 2011) that 'The old, gold standard of positive psychology was disproportionately tied to mood, the form of happiness that the ancients snobbily, but rightly, considered vulgar' (p. x). The ancients he was considering were, presumably, Socrates and Aristotle, as the title of his book, *Flourish*, refers to Aristotle's criterion of the good life that we have already considered in Chapter 1.

Seligman no longer thinks that the measure of a good life is happiness, but life satisfaction. He still thinks that a happy life may satisfy some people, but that others will feel more satisfied if they are engaged with life, have a meaningful life, accomplish the goals they have set their heart on or have positive relationships. We will come back to this more recent view when we consider life satisfaction in a later section. Despite Seligman's change of heart, research into and application of the positive psychology approach continues unabatedly.

Measuring positive feelings

Psychologists have asked people repeatedly during the course of a day ('experience sampling', this is called) how they are feeling 'now', and shown that happiness varies throughout the day with the lowest point being reached in students (Csikszentmihalyi & Hunter, 2003) when they are on their own (we discuss the link between positive feelings and socializing later in this chapter) and in older people when they are particularly inactive (Oerlemans et al., 2011).

Psychologists are therefore all too aware, like the philosophers discussed in Chapter 1, that feeling happy is a fleeting thing. This is a common problem for psychologists who use the distinction of 'state' and 'trait' to deal with it. States are short-tem; traits are persistent inclinations towards one state. Trait happiness, however, turns out not to be recognizable as happiness but as something more like enjoyment of other people's company, or extraversion (Verduyn & Brans, 2012).

Some of the variation in feelings can be reduced by averaging happiness ratings over the whole day. However, experience sampling is quite a time-consuming process. So an alternative is to ask people how happy they were 'yesterday' (Kahneman et al., 2004). This 'day reconstruction method' is used in the UK's current 'Measuring National Well-being' surveys.

Self-reported positive feelings are not the only indication of happiness. It is claimed that happiness can be demonstrated on fMRI although the principal authors of this hypothesis now seem to have changed their minds (Light, Coan, Frye, et al., 2009). Other indicators that have been used in psychological research have been quality of sleep, smiling frequency (especially spontaneous smiling involving the eyes), ratings made by friends of a person's happiness and the frequency of positive words used in speech or writing.

James Pennebaker has developed a means of automatically counting the frequency of different classes of words in text, including positive feeling words: the Linguistic and Inquiry Word Count (LIWC). Word classes counted by LIWC have had surprising predictive ability and other measures of positive emotion words have shown correlations with other measures of positivity. So Facebook's decision to adapt the LIWC (as the Facebook Gross National Happiness Index) and use it to rate the positivity of Facebook postings must have seemed a no-brainer. So many people use Facebook to make regular status updates that these seem like a certain source of information about how people are feeling. However, when the results of the LIWC are compared with self-ratings of happiness (Wang et al., 2014), the correlation is negative rather than positive. What you say about how you feel is, if anything, the opposite of how you feel. The authors of this particular study discuss several reasons – including limitations in automatic text processing – but raise the interesting possibility that reading lots of very upbeat status reports from other people, to which one politely replies positively, might actually induce a lower mood in oneself. I consider this later in the chapter when we consider 'relative affect'.

Happiness is only one kind of positive feeling. Other positive emotions include pride or self-confidence, contentment, affection, pleasurable anticipation, and satisfaction. Psychologists, like philosophers, have tended to concentrate purely on the positivity of these emotions, leaving aside their specific qualities. Some psychologists suggest that all of these, along with summary measures of happy feelings, should be bundled together in one composite measure of subjective well-being. However, not all of these feelings are likely to be predictive of long-term well-being. Pride, for example, can lead to an over-estimate of how much other people value you. As the aphorism says, 'pride comes before a fall'.

Positive psychologists often make the same distinction as philosophers between 'hedonic' happiness or reward and 'eudaimonic' happiness. Positive psychologists aim for increases in eudaimonic happiness. They are not mere hedonists. Hedonic happiness is feeling happy, now: going shopping, having a good time at a club, and so on. Eudaimonic happiness has been defined in one study as the happiness of doing good or 'engaging in inherently meaningful behaviours'. In this diary study, doing good resulted in the participants noting greater well-being in their diaries the following day than if they had had fun the previous day (Steger et al., 2008). Eudaimonic happiness, but not hedonic happiness, has been found in another study to correlate with biological markers taken to be an indication of health (Ryff et al., 2004).

Flow

Seligman sometimes puts the origins of positive psychology down to a chance meeting on holiday with a psychology colleague, Mihalyi Csikszentmihalyi. Csikszentmihalyi had also been interested in living life to the full, but, rather than concentrating on positive affect, he had been working on a quality of full absorption in a task or an experience that seemed to be going particularly smoothly and enjoyably that he termed 'flow'. The philosopher and philanthropist Lord Russell had also described this as the secret of happiness in his early 20th-century book on happiness, although he called it 'zest' and cautioned that one could pig out on flow too (Russell, 1968 (1930)).

Flow is a quality of activity that does not require much introspection. It might not be associated with strong feelings at the time, but rather afterwards the sense of flow during the activity would be what one would look back on as the enjoyable aspect. Some people, when asked about their most enjoyable experiences, might even name those that they remembered to have 'flowed'. But others might name a very difficult and poorly flowing activity that, even so and after great effort, they brought to a conclusion.

Flow experiences may also convert us from feeling negative to feeling positive. I will come back to this aspect of flow when we consider the area that positive psychology has made most contribution to – how to increase positive feelings deliberately.

Do states matter at all?

The emphasis so far has been on the less fleeting positive feelings, or rather moods, like satisfaction or content, rather than feelings themselves. But an earlier generation of humanistic psychologists was interested in extreme states, which could be transient but still left lastingly effective memories. Maslow (1968), for example, argued that 'peak experiences' linger in the memory and give us the sense of having a valuable life. Other psychologists have studied experiences that are so awful that, even when they are completely over, they leave a person hardly able to have any positive feelings again. Janoff-Bulman (1992) argues that extreme negative feelings change our perception of the world, and perhaps this is true of positive feelings too. Peak experiences are perhaps as important to our perception of life having meaning as extreme negative feelings are in making us feel that we have lost our sense of security of living in a good world.

Increasing positive feelings

Possibly the most popular, but also most divisive, aspect of positive psychology is the notion that we can deliberately increase our positive feelings at the expense of our negative ones. Proponents say that this is no different from increasing one's health by abstaining from junk foods or taking regular exercise. Opponents say that feelings that are artificially enhanced are potentially self-deceptive. Like putting on rose-tinted spectacles, they distance us from the world around us by substituting a false image for the real thing.

Van Deurzen (2009) has marshalled the arguments against focusing on happiness as the main goal of life, but, for those for whom it is the priority, positive psychology has systematized methods to increase it without any increase in motivation to be happy. Physiological studies on which areas of the brain are active during an experience show that the more active the area of the brain over the eyes (the orbitofrontal cortex), the more pleasure is prolonged and the more rewarding the experience (Light, 2009). This area of the brain is also activated by contagious emotion, and on the left side particularly, by thinking about how oneself or another person is thinking ('theory of mind') (Light, Coan, Zahn-Waxler, et al., 2009). It is probably a common feature of many of these methods that they stimulate reflection on the pleasure that we receive from an experience (Light, Coan, Frye, et al., 2009) and by thinking about it, we amplify it. What the brain is doing is only an approximate guide to what the mind is doing, but it is striking that these two principles – being more attentive or mindful of positive experiences, and acknowledging the good in others – underpin many positive psychology interventions.

The gratitude exercise is an example: think about someone who did you a favour, write a letter explaining what it was they did and then deliver it personally, as a surprise. This, its originators showed (Seligman et al., 2005), results in a prolonged increase in happiness although a later study has shown that it is only effective for some people. In others, who are naturally gloomy, the gratitude exercise may worsen their mood (Sergeant & Mongrain, 2011). Seligman et al. also evaluated two other exercises that were found to increase subjective well-being: writing one's own obituary and thinking about three positive events that had happened during the day. Like the gratitude exercise, these other exercises encourage a person to spend more time rehearsing a positive emotion. Focusing on a positive emotion seems to increase the amount of pleasure, or reward, that one gets. Another commonly used positive psychology intervention is 'savouring': thinking about a good feeling and following a procedure to ensure that one really relishes it. Focusing on the here and now, another intervention, may also be a way of increasing reward.

Focusing on the here and now is one of the principle components of 'mindfulness', another intervention commonly used by positive psychology practitioners, although its origins are in meditation techniques developed by Buddhist and Hindu monks. One effect of this might be to reduce rumination about negatives, rather than increase the focus on positives. However, regular users report an increase in well-being. Positive memories can also be savoured, although depressed people find it difficult to remember that they ever had any positive experiences (Weiser, 2012).

Imagining, and writing about, a positive future and naming one's 'signature strengths' – things that one is unusually good at – and developing them are both also tried and tested methods of enhancing well-being.

Limits to positive psychology

Positive psychology has re-introduced an emphasis on people choosing to live their lives in 'good' ways. Not morally good – that is the domain of the spiritual, which we discuss in Chapter 7 – but living life so as to enhance one's well-being. Positive psychology does not assume that one should do this at the expense of other people. It recognizes that other people have so much impact on our own lives that well-being requires that we take account of others. But it assumes that we cannot control other people's actions, only our own. So its starting point is the question, 'How can we cultivate our feelings so that well-being is enhanced?' This is, in many ways, a return to Aristotle, who asked of himself a similar question well over 2000 years ago, as I discussed in Chapter 1.

Positive psychology is upbeat and is both responsible and fun. So what could there be to say against it? Well, we can think of a few of its limitations.

First, does it fully take account of other people? Other people are certainly taken account of, but perhaps as a prop for our own well-being rather than being fully recognized as agents in themselves (I have already considered this in my commentary above). We come back to this in Chapter 8, but for now let's just say that it focuses, like many other self-help approaches, on the self, and not on our relationships or our family or the neighbours.

Second, positive psychology, understandably, focuses on the positive. It could easily be inferred from this that negative feelings are bad, that they are failings of our ability to be positive. Positive psychology may therefore reinforce the already prevailing idea that happy people are successful people. This is true empirically, as is the link between success and happiness. No one is always successful nor successful in every sphere of activity.

But the positive psychology message might be misinterpreted to mean that anyone can be happy if they are one of life's winners. If one is not – and as we have said, no one is always a winner – there is a temptation to pretend that one is, to feign happiness. So one limit to positive psychology is the extent to which it encourages people to deceive others, and themselves, about their own, true, level of well-being. We constantly live with examples of this. We are shown a world of celebrity, of glitz, glamour and smiles and may even believe it, even though we also read of the extreme stresses of celebrity life. Celebrities conspire to hide this suffering and suffer even more as a result.

Not all negative feelings result from errors in thinking. In fact, the evidence is that when we are weighing ourselves up, most people choose feeling good about themselves over the accurate self-assessment that carries with it negative feelings of disappointment or regret (Beer, 2007).

Nor are negative feelings to be avoided. We have them for good reasons. The first, and most obvious, is that negative feelings are important in life. Getting angry may lead to beneficial changes, not just for us but even for the people we get angry with. Sadness is an appropriate reaction to loss, by which we pay tribute to the value of what we have lost and give ourselves a breathing space in which to reorganize our lives. Even feelings like envy, jealousy, regret, guilt and shame have important social functions. They are problematic if they occupy too much of our time or attention, or if they become too intense. But wishing them, or thinking them, away is harmful. There is one psychiatric disorder, hypomania, in which positive feelings become intensified beyond the usual. Positive psychology might suggest that this is desirable. It's difficult to test people in this state as they are usually unwilling to fit in with another person's agenda. But people with a tendency towards mania who are given positive, negative and neutral films to watch are less tolerant of the negative films and become more irritable watching them than controls (Gruber et al., 2008). Positive feelings may therefore make people less tolerant of others who are feeling bad.

Feeling bad undoubtedly may have a bad effect. Depression causes persistently negative feelings, and the World Health Organization considers that depression is the greatest cause of disability and death in 18- to 44-year-olds worldwide. Despite claims to the contrary, there is little evidence that serious disabling depression can be rectified by positive psychology. As we shall see in the next section, at a certain point persistently low mood seems to trap people and no amount of cheering up works. One reason for this may be that being positive requires that ill-defined thing, 'mental energy' or effort (Kron et al., 2010). Commonsense psychology recognizes this. Recalcitrant teenagers who refuse to socialize with their parents are often told to 'make an effort. You'll feel better if you do'. Effort of the kind required draws on wellsprings of which little is known. There is, as I indicated in Chapter 2, a link with dopamine and a link, too, with practice at self-control. People with ADHD are less able to make this kind of effort. There is also an important link with agency and the perception that one has charge over one's life (Abel & Frohlich, 2012). Agency increases with higher status (Cheng et al., 2010). So, social status, including the status that one is born into, is not something under a person's immediate control. The positive psychology message seems directed at people of high status: people who have the resources and determination to change their life circumstances. But this may come down to good fortune in the end, and may not at all be about knowing the secrets of feeling positive (Thoits, 2006).

Positive psychology requires an optimistic view of life and relationships. But how much of this is illusion? Is life really worthwhile? Are friends really as caring or uncritical as they say? It would be nice to think so, and that feeling positive about oneself goes hand in hand with being more accurate about one's judgements of such things. But the evidence may be against this. Illusions about oneself, and one's importance in the grand scheme of things, do not reduce well-being – rather, they enhance it – but they do diminish the accuracy of our judgements about our own worth (Brookings & Serratelli, 2006).

The limits of positive psychology interventions have not been mapped. It is normal with new methods in psychology that they are considered to be substantial improvements on previous interventions, simply because they are later developments. So far there is little evidence of the long-term value of making oneself feel happier. However, one study suggests that the effect is no greater than making oneself more active (Mazzucchelli et al., 2010).

Clinical psychology

Negative feelings

There are as many nuances of negative feelings as there are of positive feelings. We may feel wistful nostalgia, regret, compassionate sadness, and so on. To simplify things for our discussion, we will use the same technique as we did for happiness. Happiness, as we discussed, is linked to a characteristic facial expression, the smile. One definition of positive emotions might therefore be that they are the family, or clade, of emotions all linked by their association with an increased likelihood of smiling, and a positive feeling is our experience of having a positive emotion. If we consider other facial expressions as linking feelings in clades, then we can ask ourselves which facial expressions are associated with more pain than pleasure. Clearly, sadness is, and so is fear, as both have characteristic and probably genetically determined facial expressions (Ekman, 2009). Disgust may or may not be a negative emotion, depending on whether or not we are disgusted with ourselves, but it also has a characteristic facial expression and therefore stands for a 'clade' of emotions. Anger, too, may or may not be negative, again depending on whether or not we are angry with ourselves. Surprise, on the other hand, does not appear to have a universal expression (Schützwohl & Reisenzein, 2012), but, like guilt, it is a derivative of fear.

Psychologists have sometimes used other fundamental criteria to produce families of emotion. An important one in the history of emotions has been the tendency to approach or avoid; another is the type of autonomic arousal involved. Increased sympathetic activity is particularly associated with anger or anxiety, often said to share a similar fight or flight response. Sadness and disgust involve increased vagal tone with slowing of the heart and nausea (people may die from being shamed), but these autonomic patterns are not clear-cut and are not emotion-specific.

Most of the research in clinical psychology has ignored the full range of negative emotions (Tantam, 1993) to focus on the 'dysphorias': anxiety or fear and depression or sadness. Anger and irritability are often taken to be consequences of dysphoria.

I have already argued that it is not always appropriate or helpful to try to do without even these unpleasant emotions. Many years ago, the psychologist Irving Janis, argued that exposure to stress (I will say more about stress in Chapter 4) might act like exposure to a vaccine. Stress 'inoculates' against future stress by enhancing our ability to deal with it (Janis, 1983). Independent studies suggest that this does work (Saunders et al., 1996). Janis's use of the term inoculation seems exactly right, because inoculation of a vaccine only works if the bug in the vaccine is killed or at least unable to cause an infection. Stress, too, is like that. If we are inoculated with a stress that overwhelms us, it does not help us but leaves us weakened. Adversity that defeats us does not increase our resilience but, if we overcome it, we are stronger for it (Seery et al., 2010). 'What does not kill you, makes you stronger', wrote Nietzsche. But some stresses do kill you or at least your ability to rise above them.

Why do people stay unhappy?

Positive psychologists argue that increasing happiness can increase the likelihood that a person will become a happy person. This is because feeling happy is rewarding. It is nice to feel happy. Increasing the frequency of happiness increases rewards, and that may be enough for a person to become happy, so long as their ongoing life provides an adequate source of reward on an everyday basis. It usually does, as happy people live in a happy world, or at least a world that affords them happiness. If, as Bentham argued and as some psychologists still argue (Huppert & So, 2013), negative feelings are on a continuum with positive feelings, then reducing negative feelings will have a comparable effect to increasing positive ones. So the clinical psychologists who reduce depression or anxiety are having a comparable effect to that of the positive psychologist, but by pushing the hedonic balance into the happy sector not by increasing positive feelings but by reducing negative ones.

Hedonic balance rests on habituation: neither positive nor negative emotions persist but, like a set of scales that has a weight taken off it, swing back to the balance point. As already mentioned in Chapter 1, the balance point is not zero. It is, for most people, on the positive side, so that most people are generally happy although some may be generally unhappy. In support of hedonic balance theory, it has been noted that even extremely rewarding events, like winning big on the lottery, do not give lasting happiness. Inversely, people who have suffered painful experiences or losses may 'bounce back' (Brickman et al., 1978).

Until they bounce back, people are vulnerable, perhaps as much from too much happiness as from too much sadness. Philosophers have, in the past, counselled people in both conditions to be careful. Lottery winners, for example, often pay for their short-term good fortune by long-term disaster. People who have suffered a severe reverse in life may never recover.

There are several reasons why negative emotions may persist, and even become self-sustaining. People may be targeted by other people wanting to exploit their vulnerability. Decision making may deteriorate under the influence of intense emotion. But perhaps most significantly, a massive emotional response may provoke persistent and undermining comparisons. People who have won the lottery may find that ordinary happy events seem insignificant, and therefore unrewarding, in relation to the lottery win. Winning a moderate amount may have a less damaging effect than winning an enormous amount or a small amount that makes one wish one had won more (Gardner & Oswald, 2007). People who have suffered a great loss may spend a lot of time comparing their present situation to the one they had before their loss (Brickman et al., 1978). Many of the interventions to foreshorten low mood may work on these comparison processes and not on mood at all, by recreating a future focus via the instillation of hope.

Longing

A politician or philanthropist – or, as we have seen, an economist – may put their efforts, and will encourage us to put ours, into making everyone's world a better place, with greater security and less economic inequality, so that everyone has the resources that they need. However, political conservatives do not necessarily agree with this. They focus on the responsibilities that each of us has to make something of our lives. This view easily slides into thinking that people who have a preponderance of negative experiences are 'negative people', who have unrealistic needs for reward. This is one of the many stigmatizing views that people take of the expression of 'negative' emotions: that it is selfish or simply the consequence of wanting too much out of life without putting enough back.

The psychologist's contribution is to consider how to help individuals find more rewards in their present lives, without longingly waiting for a future world of a better kind. Longing in this way, without acting on the longing, just makes negative feelings worse.

Some of the earliest epidemiological studies in psychiatry were undertaken just after the Second World War. The rates of depression and anxiety – up to 90% in Manhattan and rural Canada – found in them astounded many researchers. These studies were ridiculed at the time, and the next generation of epidemiologists often incorporated some measure of severity, sometimes called 'caseness', into their studies. 'Caseness' meant: 'Would a person with this degree of depression or anxiety normally consider going to a doctor for treatment? And would the doctor accept that they had a disorder?' The proportion of people with depression or anxiety, when this cut-off is applied, drops very considerably. Similarly, many people in the general population report that they are in less than perfect health on any particular day, but only a minority of them are 'ill'. We are going to consider people with cases of mental and physical disorder in the next chapter. In this chapter, we consider the much larger group of people who do not consider that they are ill, but do consider that they are unhappy or bothered by worries and fears.

Bouncing back: resilience

Balls that bounce are essential to social games like tennis, football, cricket and baseball. But balls that do not bounce back are used in games, too, although these are games of positioning: croquet, petanque and bowls, for example. Resilience in psychological terms is 'bounciness': the ability to recover from some adversity and bounce back from the shock to one's former state. Having positive feelings about other aspects of one's life is an important element in bouncing back (Cohn et al., 2009), perhaps because positive feelings encourage social exploration, according to the 'broaden and build' approach of Fredrickson (Fredrickson, 2004). Bouncing back means maintaining social involvement and continuing the game. Resilience too means restoring the status quo and this often means continuing to function socially as before. What if one cannot bounce back? What is the future then? In bowls, if one player knocks the previous player's wood away from the jack, one riposte is to try to reposition the jack. Is there an equivalent psychologically? I would say that there is. If other people consistently knock you away from the goal that you are aiming at, perhaps you need to move your goal and not make more and more strenuous, but frustrated, attempts to reach that goal. Once, I played croquet with a close friend, who was a very good player. Croquet is a devilish game because you are allowed to knock the other player's balls about in order to gain extra turns. In fact, it is hardly a social game at all. One player may go and do something else whilst the other player is having their turn, as it is painful to see all your carefully laid-out positioning undone. On this occasion, there was nowhere else to go, so I watched as my balls were being driven hither and thither, but it became obvious that driving my balls away was more important to my opponent than winning. Both of us were aiming to get to the finishing post, but keeping me away from the post seemed more important for my friend than getting there himself. It was a crushing, and humiliating, defeat. But it taught me one thing: that competing with my friend for the same goals in life was going to be the end of our friendship. A repeat croquet match was out of the question, in other words. Any future friendship would have to be based on respect for each other's different objectives in life and not comparing our success on any shared goals. Resilience is not the only way to deal with reverses. Sometimes, one has to start again but go in a different direction.

I will come back to this perspective when we consider how psychotherapists look at things (Chapter 8). Psychologists tend to consider just the bouncing back kind of coping with adversity, partly because theirs is a prosocial perspective, and partly because the emphasis of psychology is on overcoming and mastery.

How can negative feelings be used to increase health or well-being?

Negative feelings are, by definition, states we want to change. They motivate us to change. But the range of possible changes that we can make encompasses measures that may increase or decrease well-being, and may improve or lead to a deterioration in our health. Other people may be influential in which change strategy we pick, as may our own experience and what we have learnt during our lives about what works and what does not. Some would say that our choices are entirely determined by these influences, but I do not think so. I think that even in the most over-determined circumstances, we do have a choice. Everyone has creativity in their mental make-up. Each of us can take a step along an unexpected path. Some people might say – do say when I am discussing the existential approaches to which these ideas are central – 'What if a person is in solitary confinement? What choices do they have then?' I would point to Nelson Mandela's experience or that of Victor Frankl (Frankl, 1963) in an earlier generation (there is more about Victor Frankl in Chapter 8).

Making changes in one's life presupposes that one knows what changes to make and that one has the power to make them. Psychologists have looked at both of these issues.

Health psychology

Knowing how to change

Psychologists sometimes prioritize knowledge over emotion, and things that we can demonstrate over things that we know instinctively. We all rely on feelings about what to do to some degree, but these are difficult to explain or put into words. So recommendations to other people on how they might change their lives in response to negative feelings have tended to emphasize explicit strategies or plans. Possibly one of the most comprehensive approaches to planning what to do about negative feelings is 'coping'. Coping is an old term for two contenders meeting in a battle or fight, called a 'coping'. This meaning passed on to contending with a difficulty, but it was first put forward as a strategy, as something one could become skilled at, by psychoanalytically orientated psychotherapists in the mid-20th century. The psychologist Richard Lazarus gave coping its current shape by emphasizing the importance of appraisal and of thought patterns or 'cognitions' in shaping emotional responses to stress (we say more about appraisal and cognitions below). He and his co-workers tied ways of appraising and ways of thinking about stress together in a range of coping strategies, some of which were provocatively contrary to commonsense psychology, for example denying there is a problem can often be the most effective coping strategy (Lazarus & Folkman, 1984). Lazarus and Folkman identified several coping strategies, but many more have been proposed since then. Coping skills or coping strategies are often cited in self-help or self-improvement approaches to negative feelings.

Nudging

One of the more striking aspects of human behaviour is our propensity to know what is good for us and choose to do the opposite. I have already mentioned the ancient Greek ideas about this, which were based on akrasia. This was translated by English and Scottish 19th-century theologians and philosophers as weakness of will but actually meant powerlessness. Children who are described as 'wilful' do not grow up into adults with a lot of 'will power'. So the concept of 'will' does not seem to fit with the Victorian idea that some people have more will power than others. Akrasia includes other kinds of power, including the possibility that our power to change is diminished by external circumstances. Health psychologists are often in the business of helping people switch to a healthier lifestyle, and are well aware of these issues.

Health psychologists increasingly take account of external factors rather than simply appealing to will power. Michie et al.'s (2011) 'behaviour change wheel' is an example of this (see Figure 3.1).

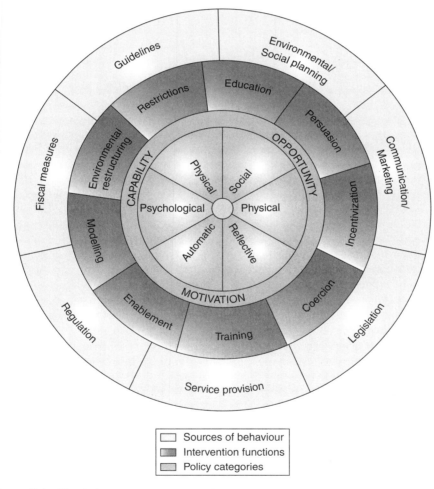

Figure 3.1 The behaviour change wheel

Source: Michie et al., 2011

The inner circle of the behaviour change wheel accounts for external factors in its recognition of the importance of opportunity, recognizes that people might lack the capability to change and focuses on motivation as what needs to be targeted to bring about change. The starting point for change is a measure of attitudes and intentions, as well as behaviours to identify a target for intervention. The theory of planned behaviour is well known (Ajzen & Madden, 1986). Once a target behaviour has been identified – say, going to the gym or giving up smoking – a behaviour change technique can be chosen to take account of the target behaviour and of the constraints, many of which are shown in Figure 3.1, on the possibility of change. Health psychologists distinguish between identifying a target behaviour – for which the theory of planned behaviour was designed – and choosing an intervention. Michie and colleagues (2013) have come up with a list of 93 behaviour change techniques for a health psychologist to change another person's motivation. The list, like the assessments in the theory of planned behaviour, is largely cognitive. The theory of planned behaviour works for some people reasonably well, but not at all for others (Hobbs et al., 2013). One possible explanation is that it does not account for emotional choices, which may include those that are destructive and likely to lead to reduced well-being.

Appraisal theory, cognitive therapy and behavioural therapy

Another approach to behaviour change is to consider that behaviour is a way of dealing with a situation, a way of 'coping'. One element of Lazarus's coping theory was that negative feelings are the result of interpreting an event or a happening as a threat, a challenge, a loss or some other reason for negative feeling. A cognitive step of 'appraisal' came before and influenced the emotional reaction of depression or anxiety. It has been suggested that we are more or less inclined to do this, depending on 'schemata' or 'emotional scripts' that have been created by personal experience that has been 'wired in'. Appraisals may also be influenced by current feelings. People with a tendency to anxiety are more likely to see threats. People who are currently anxious are also more likely to see threats. Indeed, it may be argued that the function of anxiety is to be alert to threats and ready to deal with them.

Coping theory belongs to a thread of Stoic approaches to well-being, in which well-being is seen to depend on the mastery of the emotions by the intellect. However, coping may be generalized to emotions, too. Re-defining anxiety from being pathology to having value in scanning for and responding to threats might be said, by extension, to be another way of 'coping with it'. This was the existentialist approach championed by Rollo May (May, 1950).

Another approach is to encourage a person to alter their appraisals, perhaps by changing their bias towards threat. This approach implies that the appraisal is somehow faulty or 'not adaptive', to use a term that was introduced to be 'value-free'. But, in fact, values are inseparable from judgements about negative feelings. We cannot but consider whether persisting negative feelings are misleading us, or whether they are alerting us to something important, something we should not neglect. Encouraging a person to change their appraisal is only justifiable if we assume that their current appraisal is self-deceptive in some way. One anxiety that we have about the uptake of positive psychology, or indeed coping theory, is that greater credence will be given to the idea that negative feelings can be assumed to be a consequence of a negative world view or some other kind of failing.

Connor-Smith and Flachsbart (Connor-Smith & Flachsbart, 2007) suggest that coping skills fall into several families (see Table 3.1). A few are about coping with the negative emotion itself, for example by 'acting out': throwing things, getting angry

Table 3.1 Types of coping strategy

Coping Code	Definition
Negative Emotion Focused	Emotion regulation and expression strategies that suggest loss of control (e.g., hitting, throwing objects), distress (e.g., crying, yelling, self-blame) or hostility towards others.
Mixed Emotion Focused	Responses to emotional distress involving a mix of controlled and uncontrolled emotion regulation and expression strategies.
Engagement Coping	Broad category of approach-orientated responses directed toward the stressor or one's reactions to the stressor.
Primary Control	Active attempts to control or change a bad situation or one's emotional reaction to the situation.
Problem Solving	Active attempts to resolve a stressor through planning, generation of possible solutions, logical analysis and evaluation of options, implementing solutions, and staying organized and on task.
Instrumental Support	Problem-focused social support, including seeking help, resources, or advice about possible solutions to problems.
Emotional Support	Emotion-focused social support, including seeking comfort, empathy, and closeness with others.
Mixed Social Support	A combination of instrumental and emotional support.
Emotional Regulation	Active attempts to decrease negative emotions through controlled use of strategies such as relaxation or exercise, or modulating expressions of emotion to ensure that feelings are expressed at an appropriate time in a constructive manner.
Secondary Control	Attempts to adapt to a stressor to create a better fit between the self and the environment.
Distraction	Taking a temporary break from a stressful situation by engaging in an enjoyable activity. Distraction does NOT involve attempts to avoid or deny problems.

(Continued)

Table 3.1 (Continued)

Coping Code	Definition
Cognitive Restricting	Finding a more positive or realistic way to think about a bad situation, looking on the bright side, identifying benefits arising from the situation (e.g., personal growth) or finding a humorous side to the stressor.
Acceptance	Coming to terms with aspects of the stressor that can't be changed, learning to live with the stressors or one's limitations, developing a sense of understanding.
Religious Coping	Having faith in God, praying about the stressor, participating in religious services or activities.
Broad Disengagement	Broad category of responses oriented away from the stressor or one's reactions to the stressor. Historically, broad disengagement scales have included distraction, substance use and symptoms of distress.
Narrow Disengagement	Disengagement responses excluding distraction, substance use and symptoms of distress.
Avoidance	Attempts to avoid the problem, reminders of the problem, thoughts of the problem or emotions related to the problem.
Denial	Active attempts to deny or forget about a problem, to hide your emotional response from yourself or others.
Wishful Thinking	Hoping to be magically rescued from the situation or for the situation to disappear, fantasizing about unlikely outcomes, wishing that you or the situation were radically different.
Withdrawal	Intentionally isolating one's self, spending time alone, choosing not to share problems or emotions with others.
Substance Use	Use of alcohol, nicotine or illegal drugs for the specific purpose of coping with stress.

Source: Connor-Smith & Flachsbart, 2007, Relations between personality and coping: a meta-analysis. *Journal of Personality and Social Psychology*, 93(6), 1080–1107.

with people, carrying on. These uncontrolled coping strategies may or may not be combined with more controlled strategies: counting to 10 when one is angry, taking controlled breaths with anxiety, and so on. Most coping strategies are directed towards dealing with the stimulus that has caused the negative emotion. Some require engaging with the cause of negative feelings, whilst others involve disengagement. Connor-Smith and Flachsbart (2007) suggest that engagement may mean trying to overcome the cause of the negative feeling (primary control) or adapting more effectively to it (secondary control).

Schema theory has also led to a focus on the part that unconscious processing plays in the consequences of appraisal. The cognitive elements of appraisal normally happen too

quickly to allow for conscious consideration. We see a soldier coming down the
we feel fear, without being aware that in the process we have looked at the person's
correctly identified it as an army uniform, inferred that the approaching person is a
and triggered images of fighting, killing or rape that our own personal experience or media
reports may have created in our minds in association with the image of a soldier. (We are
assuming here the perspective of a civilian with no experience of actual soldiers. Soldiers
will obviously have a very different schema of each other, as may their wives, parents or
children, and civil servants in the Ministry of Defence.) Having seen the soldier and felt
that *frisson* of fear, we may tell ourselves that our reaction is inappropriate, we may focus
on the soldier's youth and air of timidity, we may search visually for whether or not he or
she has a weapon, and so on. The appraisal triggers further thoughts and mental action or
'cognitions'. Some of these are automatic but some are under our control. For example, we
may stop looking at the uniform and focus on the face or eyes of the soldier, which will
immediately make them more like a person and less like an impersonal threat, and we can
remind ourselves to do this. Surprisingly, we can even overcome neurological impairments
in this way. In one case study, a woman with a very small tumour in one part of her brain
(the amygdala) lost the normal propensity to look at other people's faces when interacting
with them. Consequently, she often made mistakes about what other people were feeling.
When she was asked to make a conscious effort to look at another person's face and especially their eyes, she did so and her ability to pick up on their feelings improved; but she
quickly forgot to do so (Adolphs et al., 2005). This is one potential limitation of cognitive
approaches. They need to be maintained by an effort of will until they become habitual.

Changing habits of emotional response ('conditioned responses') was the rationale of
behaviour therapy. First, old habits had to be unlearned and this could often be done by
quite simple procedures. For example, a fear of spiders can be effectively unlearned in three
hours by increasing levels of exposure to a spider (Ost, 1996). Of course, this must be a
harmless spider. Exposure to one that bites (not common in spiders) will simply increase
fear. The longer it takes to learn new habits, the longer they generally last, but a sufficiently
devastating exerience can erase them. People being people, thinking is always involved in
changing habits. For example, exposure therapy for spider phobia is not effective if the person being exposed is thinking the whole time, 'This spider is harmless, but that's not true
of the spiders at home'. Hence, cognitive and behavioural elements are usually combined.

Some habits are not mediated by conscious thought. Habits of going to bed early,
having a hot drink when one wakes in the night and drinking a lot of caffeine in the day
are associated with insomnia. Even waking up in the night is associated with insomnia
the next night, but especially so if one becomes wide awake, for example because one
turns the television on. Less obviously, spending a long time lying in bed and putting
off doing tasks that require energy can also become habits that reinforce the low mood
that originally triggered them. 'Behavioural' activation may be associated with a reduction in negative feelings and an increase in well-being because breaking the habit of
inaction reduces the self-condemnation that goes with the habit. In fact, behavioural
activation has been found to be as effective as the most effective of the positive psychology interventions that we considered previously (Mazzucchelli et al., 2010). The effect is
not mediated by exercise. Contrary to commonsense psychology, exercise has not been

found to consistently reduce negative feelings (Lawlor & Hopker, 2001), although it may improve health. Switching from being passive to active is what improves well-being.

The power to change

Changing negative feelings, in fact changing any habits, including dispositions to particular emotional reactions or over-use of particular kinds of appraisal, is hard. It takes effort – or will, drive or determination or, to use Heidegger's term, resoluteness or even, to cite Tillich, 'courage'. Will, however, as I have already noted, is not just an inner resource. One needs to feel positive to change a negative feeling (Kashdan et al., 2011) and one also needs to feel in tune with one's values.

The Victorians were fascinated by will and its 'power', and Freud's dynamic theory of how the mind works was intended to be an explanation of how it arose. Will has dropped out of academic psychology, although not out of commonsense psychology. Its demise was probably due to it explaining too much. Ideas that seem to explain everything, like 'life force' or 'destiny', often turn out to be dead ends because if everything is explained then nothing that is particularly relevant to the situation being considered is explained. But there is clearly something that means that one person takes on a difficult personal change and completes it, whilst another person gives up. There is a surprisingly simple measure of it – grip strength. A strong handshake, measured by a dynamometer, predicts mental and physical health 50 years hence. Perhaps it is an interaction between the nature of the task and the dispositions of the person. Perhaps it is timing or some dramatic upheaval that makes change possible. Challenges to pre-existing, fixed values due to changes in circumstances may be liberating as well as fear-provoking. The psychologist Albert Bandura, thought that change was due to self-belief, leading to what he called 'self-efficacy'.

Self-efficacy may not be an attribute of the self at all, at least not wholly. It may be a reflection of social relationships, as assessed by social status and also by social isolation. Status, or some corollary of status, may even have an epigenetic effect, turning some genes on, for example those influencing intelligence (Tucker-Drob et al., 2011). Low status and high social isolation independently increase ill health, particularly among young males (Heritage, 2009). Low status is also associated with a persistence in negative feelings (Murphy et al., 1991), possibly mediated by the effective levels of one neurotransmitter, serotonin (Kiser et al., 2012), the transmitter that is the main target of the 'new' SSRI antidepressants. Social relationships provide opportunities for social reward, and social status means that others are more likely to be willing to provide practical help. But there may be more to it than that. It is possible for life to become so repeatedly difficult that eventually a person gives up and does not even try anymore to overcome their negative feelings. This state was once termed learned helplessness, but nowadays it is more common to call it a state of 'defeat'. Defeat blocks the wish to seek happiness, as well as the wish to escape from negative feelings (Gilbert et al., 2002). Defeat is often associated with a feeling of hopelessness.

Another factor that may lock a person into a state of negative feeling, and therefore low well-being, is that of feeling 'trapped'. Entrapment occurs when any course of action leads to an increase in negative feeling. Even though there may be a course of action that can be expected to lead to positive feelings in the long run, the intervening negative feelings are just too great a bar to taking that course. Entrapment is often associated with feelings of helplessness. People get entrapped in failing marriages, in decaying neighbourhoods and in dead-end jobs. It may just not be possible to find the energy to get out of negative feelings, or to find short-term methods of changing them, which, as we will show in the next chapter, are often just those behaviours that may lead to poorer health outcomes.

'I've been down so long, it looks like up to me'

This is the title of a book written by Richard Farina, the brother-in-law of singer and activist Joan Baez. Farina was a well-known folk singer himself and wrote the book whilst studying at Cornell University. The book is written in the first person and describes someone who is lost in drugs, dreads being drafted into fighting in Vietnam and has a sense of meaninglessness. Farina was killed, riding pillion on someone else's motorbike, shortly after the first launch party for the book. The mood of the book may not have been in keeping with Farina's purposeful life, but it chimed with enough young people in the 1960s to have been turned into a film and to have given its title to popular songs.

I have chosen it because it is a graphic illustration of how negative feelings can become so much the norm in a person's world that they no longer point to a direction in which change could happen, but point paradoxically towards actions that will decrease well-being. Making it a priority to get rid of the negative feeling as soon as possible is a common feature of dealing with negative feelings in such a way as to decrease long-term well-being. The commonsense psychology term for this is 'not facing up to your feelings', but facing up to feelings is not so easy to do. The philosopher Sartre considered that we become conscious of our emotions only in order to 'magically transform' our world (Sartre, 1971). In other words, Sartre thought it impossible to hold on to strong negative feelings without trying to change the world, or at least one's perception of it, to make the feeling go away. I will consider in Chapter 8 how people twist and turn to make their world seem different from what it is. Here, we will consider some of the methods for dealing with negative feelings that have received particular attention from psychologists, noting those that lead to long-term well-being and those that do not.

Comfort

Comfort is much more of a danger when one is feeling negative than when one is feeling positive, when it is not needed. Taking comfort in what life is offering does not present any danger, but seeking comfort is like seeking happiness – it can easily distort the shape of one's life. And it can become addictive: eating sweet foods, not because one is hungry but to relieve negative feelings (Dubé et al., 2005); drinking alcohol or taking sedatives or painkillers; slumping in front of the television; watching porn or gambling on the internet – all of these offer comfort but risk perpetuating negative feelings. Rats fed cafeteria-style food have an increased transmitter in an area of the brain associated with reward (mesolimbic dopamine increased) but the ordinary laboratory chow no longer increases dopamine as it did before. The rats are only rewarded by the cafeteria-style food and this, as it turns out, makes them fat (Dubé et al., 2005). Getting hooked on the internet or drinking too much become problematic if they are persistent. But the starting point is the urgent need to get rid of negative emotion (Dallman et al., 2003) or feelings of loneliness (Troisi & Gabriel, 2011) by tasting food that has the emotional flavour of an earlier close relationship.

Ressentiment, shame and resentment

Fear and anxiety are not the only negative feelings. Anger, especially impotent anger, is a maddening emotion that almost invites the sufferer to hide it, leading to a situation to which the Danish philosopher Kierkegaard and later the German philosopher Nietzsche applied the term 'ressentiment'. The sociologist Max Scheler wrote a book about ressentiment, applying it to many 20th-century cultural problems. He defined it as:

> a self-poisoning of the mind which has quite definite causes and consequences. It is a lasting mental attitude, caused by the systematic repression of certain emotions and affects which, as such, are normal components of human nature. Their repression leads to the constant tendency to indulge in certain kinds of value delusions and corresponding value judgments. The emotions and affects primarily concerned are revenge, hatred, malice, envy, the impulse to detract, and spite. (Scheler, 1994: 45–46)

Ressentiment is a kind of false humility or, as Nietzsche called it, the morality of the slave. Shame is another negative emotion that may be hidden but, like ressentiment, it involves constant concealment and perpetuates the very negative feelings that it is intended to nullify. Hidden negative emotions lead to a conviction that one is inferior to others, and this can lead to pleasure ('Schadenfreude') at the losses of people that one judges to be superior (Leach & Spears, 2008) but also to increased negative feelings at their gains. Usually, even these negative feelings overwhelm the positive ones.

Ressentiment, and shame, may be deeply hidden under a cloak of duty, servility or dedication, but negative feelings about other people are not always buried. Many people who are confronted in their daily lives with other people's good fortune may feel angry and resentful. Some may feel envious and conclude that life is unfair. Others may look for opportunities to do harm to more fortunate others, through acts of spite or petty vandalism. These are all means to remove negative feelings, since none of them increase our own well-being in any other way. It is likely that these are universal instincts, perhaps fostered by culture to reduce social inequality, but their net effect is to perpetuate negative feelings in anyone who becomes preoccupied with their lack of achievement relative to some other person who becomes their comparator. Prolonged negative feelings and a lack of positive feelings independently and additively (Weiser, 2012) result in poorer health and earlier death. So how people add up their lives or how people compute their 'life satisfaction' has considerable implications for their well-being.

Self-esteem

Self-esteem has been traced back to 17th-century French writers and their concept of amour-propre or self-love. La Rochefoucauld's maxims have been considered one of the clearest expositions of this (Clark, 1994). La Rochefoucauld lived at the time that France was becoming the great state of Europe. He figures in military and political accounts of the period, and appears in Alexandre Dumas's fictional recreation of it, *The Three Musketeers*. His life was full of conflict. He loved another man's wife but she chose to stay with her husband. He was a Frondeur, plotting with the Queen mother against the King, but both Frondes were defeated. He was sympathetic to the Jansenists who were shortly to be hunted down and killed by their more orthodox Roman Catholic fellow citizens.

Not surprisingly, La Rochefoucauld's maxims refer frequently to conflict. He anticipated Freud by several centuries in supposing that people often act out of internal conflict, although he expressed this conflict as between the heart, of which we are unconscious, and the mind. He wrote: 'L'homme croit souvent qu'il se conduire lorsqu' il est conduit; et pendant que par son esprit tend a un but, son coeur l'entraine insensiblement a un autre' ('People often think that they are in the driving seat, even when they are driven; while they think that they are aiming at one goal, their hearts are, without their knowing it, driving them towards another one') (Maxim 43). The goal of the heart, La Rochefoucauld thought, is the love of self or, as we would now say, 'self-esteem'. This kind of love is not sexual but it is pleasurable. So we feel good about ourselves if we have high self-esteem. Honours, favours and advancement were the stuff of La Rochefoucauld's world and love for these was an important element in his conception of self-love. Self-esteem, too, is linked to the world's esteem. Loss of esteem reduces the love that is given to ourselves and we therefore seek to avoid that happening by acting to keep the esteem of others. Thomas Scheff (personal communication) has argued that this is all the concept of self-esteem amounts to, or rather that self-esteem is really measured by the unlikelihood that we will lose other people's esteem and be shamed by them. However, for La Rochefoucauld amour propre provided a more complete explanation of all human motivation, explaining how we are shaped both by the approbation of others and by our fears. For example, he thought that we act justly because we love ourselves when we are just, and that is because we love justice but only because it protects us from the injustice of others: 'L'amour de la justice n'est en la plupart des hommes que la crainte de souffrir l'injustice' ('love of justice is for most people solely [motivated by] a fear of being treated unjustly themselves') (Maxim 79).

Self-esteem, like La Rochefoucauld's amour-propre, provides a possible synthesis between positive and negative emotions as it combines both the idea of loving oneself and of being worthy of life. But the influential social psychologist, Roy Baumeister (2005), has noted that since the 1970s self-esteem has been increasingly interpreted to mean being pleased with oneself. According to this view, negative feelings are something to be banished rather than responded to. Like the influential psychotherapist Albert Ellis, he thinks that this means being easy on ourselves. This kind of self-esteem is, understandably, correlated with self-rated happiness and it is also correlated with taking initiatives, but these initiatives may include bullying other people, taking drugs or having sex at a young age – all, according to Baumeister's review, positively correlated with self-esteem.

One of the origins of the self-esteem movement was the humanistic psychology of the 1940s. This was not quite as self-centered as the picture of self-esteem that Baumeister paints. Carl Rogers thought that loving ourselves went along with 'unconditional positive regard' for other people. It is difficult though to see how any but a saint could 'unconditionally' love another person. As La Rochefoucauld put it, 'Il est du véritable amour comme de l'apparition des esprits: tout le monde en parle, mais peu de gens en ont vu' ('it is for true love as it is for seeing ghosts: everyone talks about it, but few have actually seen it') (Maxim 76). However, La Rochefoucauld was a Jansenist. He wanted to see a return to Augustinian values in the Church. He did not give up on the possibility that self-love was just a reflection of something deeper, a fundamental way of interacting not just with oneself but with the world. He could never find it, however, living as he did in a time of magnificent hedonism: 'S'il y a un amour pur et exempt du mélange de nos autres passions, c'est celui qui est caché au fond du cœur, et que nous ignorons nous-mêmes' ('If there is a pure love, unmixed by other sentiments, then this is what we hide deep in our hearts, and even forget about it ourselves'). We will consider this again from the spiritual viewpoint, when we wonder whether an individual can ever be said to be living well unless they are contributing to the thriving of all those around them.

4

The Health Worker's Viewpoint

We can introspect our state of happiness, but the feelings that go with good health are more difficult to pin down. However, as I argued in Chapter 1, we do sometimes feel good about our bodies' functioning and, if we are healthy, we can usually tell that we are once we think about it, even if we are not feeling actively fit. Self-reported health is inversely correlated with the uptake of medical care, although it also has cultural influences (O'Reilly & Rosato, 2010). If spontaneous feelings of healthiness are even more evanescent than self-consciously happy feelings, then feelings of unhealthiness are often overwhelming and harder to disregard than negative feelings.

'Holistic health' is holistic because it tackles happiness and health together. The gym and jogging culture, focusing on bodily improvement, is a twin of the positive psychology movement, focusing on emotional improvement. Health psychology has as much kinship with sports and occupational psychology, in its emphasis on improving performance, as it does with clinical psychology, which focuses on helping people minimize the pain or disability of illness. The holistic approach and the focus on growth or development rather than repair are emphasized in complementary healing practices, which often contrast themselves with allopathic, Western medicine.

Although good health and happiness are intertwined, poor health does not always lead to unhappiness, and unhappiness is not always associated with poor health. The first UK well-being survey found that 40% of people who rate their own health as bad or very bad still report medium to high levels of satisfaction with life (although this is not quite the same as happiness). On the other hand, 80% of people who rate their health as good or very good report medium to high levels of life satisfaction (Self et al., 2012) (the data for happiness were not reported).

However, it is not right to say that Western medicine has always confined itself to fire-fighting. Perhaps it is its remarkable success at this that has attracted the headlines and taken the emphasis away from the steady increase in quality of life achieved since adopting Western medicine. Western doctors, nurses and other professionals are also concerned with health promotion, and public health medicine moved at the turn of the last century from the prevention of epidemics to general improvement in public health. The founding charter of the World Health Organization in 1948 defined health as a 'positive state of physical and mental well-being' and this definition was re-asserted in the Ottawa Charter for Health Promotion issued jointly by the WHO and other health promotion organizations in 1986.

Positive health

We saw in the previous chapter that there are lots of varieties of happiness – joy, elation, contentment, and so on – and this is also true of health. We can feel vigorous and healthy, relaxed and healthy, strong and healthy, and so on. But the underlying state of health, like the underlying disposition to happiness, is unitary, in contrast to the myriad ways that we can be unhealthy.

Feeling positively healthy can be as misleading as feeling happy and joyful. Taking large doses of steroid hormones will do it for many people, but steroids turn out to have deleterious effects on health in the long term. Running or exercising a lot can also make people feel good (it has been suggested that this is because heavy exercise releases endogenous opioids), but in the long run can lead to arthritis and fractures.

Cultures have often confounded what is good for the health with ethical or moral systems that have quite different purposes. The dietary restrictions of Vedic medicine, the basis of Ayurvedic medical practices, may have begun as caste-related practices, being nothing to do with health at all. In the same vein, a list of healthy practices is attributed to the pre-Socratic philosopher Pythagoras, but not many have stood the test of time, although his absolute prohibition of beans would have been good advice for those of his followers who had a deficiency of the enzyme glucose-6-phosphate dehydrogenase (G6DP), in whom beans may cause 'favism', the destruction of red blood cells leading to anaemia (Pirmohamed, 2011).

G6DP deficiency is rare in Northern Europe (although more common in the Mediterranean area, where Pythagoras lived, if he was a historical figure), so Pythagorean rules about beans are not good general advice about health. However, there do now exist simple but universal rules that increase life expectancy, including taking moderate exercise, maintaining normal body weight, not smoking vegetable materials, using alcohol or other drugs moderately (what constitutes moderate is contested), following a full programme of vaccinations, having safe sex, ensuring good dental care and hand hygiene, partaking in a rounded diet and avoiding rotting or preserved food and saturated fats in the diet (unless one is an Inuit).

Many people lack the resources to follow these rules, whilst others do not follow them even though they have the resources. One reason is the power of cultural rules that might require unhealthy practices. Another is the placebo or comfort effect. We will argue later that a further reason may be another manifestation of the link between emotional status and health – comfort eating.

Culture and family influences on health

As I sit in my office and write, I can see birds regularly visiting our bird table. Sometimes either I or my wife will put out a new food, and we have noticed that fledglings are often fed by a mature bird with a morsel of this. This is the opposite of what happens with familiar foods, when mature birds will actively compete with fledglings for it. The literature on allo-feeding in birds is unexpectedly limited (Scheid et al., 2008), but my observations suggest that parents pass on their knowledge of what is healthy to eat to their offspring by allo-feeding. Certainly this happens in human families. Our first knowledge about the healthiness of foods comes from what our parents or carers feed us. We may revise our opinions later, but never quite rid ourselves of that hankering for nursery food, particularly when we are feeling unwell.

Family members and carers also feed us with ideas about health and what to do to increase or decrease it. Unfortunately, not all of these ideas correspond to empirical findings across cultures.

The placebo effect

The word placebo ('I will please') was written in Latin as an instruction to the dispenser by a doctor because that was the language of medical prescription. It continues to be written in Latin to conceal the fact that the placebo is assumed by the prescriber to be inert or ineffectual. Despite this lack of confidence by the prescriber, the placebo is presented as effective and, as it turns out, often is effective although it is not clear why (Colloca & Miller, 2011). However, expectancy of benefit – hope, as I called it in the last chapter – does seem to play a part (Enck et al., 2011), although, curiously, being told that something is a placebo does not seem to remove the placebo effect. The effectiveness of a placebo is shaped by therapeutic context. The enormous public spending on apparently ineffective over-the-counter medication is an expression of the confidence-inspiring nature of pharmaceutical companies' marketing. There is evidence that the size of the placebo response has been increasing in recent decades. It is probably most important in reducing the emotional distress, discomfort and pain of illness. For example, it is claimed that the placebo response now amounts to over two-thirds of the antidepressant response to medication (Rief et al., 2009). Curiously, the placebo response can still be evoked if a person knows that they are taking an inactive preparation (Kaptchuk et al., 2010).

Many families, and some cultures, have foods that constitute placebos. Many health interventions have been sanctioned by their obvious benefit as reported by patients, despite turning out to be harmless or even harmful later. The 18th-century practice of blood-letting is an example. Our own health practices are therefore influenced not just by what our families have taught us, but by how our culture – including advertising media – shapes our health beliefs and therefore our expectancies. The history of medicine is littered with examples of apparently self-evidently good health interventions that have been maintained for generations, unassailed by what would now be called 'evidence-based medicine'. Indeed, this is why evidence-based medicine was developed. Evidence in this sense is required to be controlled in some way: that is, the effect of the intervention has to be compared to the effect of no or an ineffectual intervention in a comparable group over the same time period. The best evidence comes from randomized controlled trials in which the control is a sham intervention or placebo.

What is health?

There are positive and negative interpretations of health, just as there are for happiness, as we saw in the last chapter. The negative view is that health is the absence of ill health, as expressed by symptoms or signs of disorder, disease or disability. The positive view is that being healthy means having some protection against all disease, being slower to age and having the ability to recover more quickly from injury. Age at death is used as the gold standard of health, although from the health economist's viewpoint, as we saw in Chapter 2, it might be better to use quality adjusted life years. When planning community interventions, the age of death of the average person can be estimated by the all-cause mortality rate of the population, although, in the West where individuals are living longer and longer, this is probably an under-estimate as the duration of life continues to increase.

Average age of death is an indicator of the health of the population concerned and this can be a useful measure for public health physicians and government officials. Individual longevity cannot, of course, be known until after death, which makes it unhelpful as a measure of the health of the individual who has died. However, estimates of how long a person can be expected to live, their life expectancy, can be estimated from predictors identified in longitudinal studies of comparable populations. These predictors may change with age and with the presence of co-existing disease.

Some predictors of longevity are unalterable. These include the genetic factors that account for the members of some families living longer than the members of others. The genes or gene interactions responsible for this heritability of health are being sought (Slagboom et al., 2011), often by looking at unusually long-lived populations (see below).

Other predictors of longevity can be altered by a determined person. Such predictors include weight, diet, use of drink or drugs and activity levels. We shall consider this in more detail in a separate section.

How can we measure health?

Although spontaneous feelings of health are rare, people are generally willing to rate their own health. People who answer 'poor' to a single question, e.g. 'In general, how would you rate your health?', are twice as likely to die during the follow-up period than people who answer 'excellent' to this question (DeSalvo et al., 2006). Other studies come to the same conclusion, indicating that self-rated health is a valid measure of health. Interestingly, doctors' ratings of their patients' health are half as good at predicting which of their patients will die early as those patients' self-ratings (DeSalvo & Muntner, 2011).

People rate their health according to a subjective checklist of activities, for example their ability to be at work, to exercise or to be active sexually (Winefield & Cormack, 1986). One of the standard questionnaires of health status, the short-form 36 or SF36, developed by the Rand Health Organization, is based around such a menu.

According to the conference board of Canada website (www.conferenceboard.ca/hcp/Details/Health/self-reported-health-status.aspx), surveys show that over three quarters of people in most developed countries consider that their health is 'good' or 'very good', probably using some such self-rating of activity. However, according to statistics published on the same site, life expectancy shows some marked discrepancies with these self-ratings. The Japanese, for example, rate their health as the least good of anyone in the 17 countries considered, but have the second longest life expectancy (with Hong Kong the first at the time of writing). The second most pessimistic group are the Italians, but they have the third longest life expectancy. US citizens are very close to Canadians in rating their health as the best, but have the worst life expectancy compared to citizens of the other 16 countries. (The UK does not do well on life expectancy or on self-rated health.) So self-rated health, at least in some countries, bears little relation to a commonly used measure of 'the public health'. Self-rated health correlates less and less with objective measures of health as people get older (Pinquart, 2001).

Does this mean that there is some feeling of healthiness that we can introspect? Most likely not. If we feel unhealthy, and we do not have a disorder, it is most likely that what we are picking up on in ourselves are the symptoms of depression. Depression is associated with an increased risk of death (Zheng et al., 1997) and also colours self-evaluations of health (Trentini et al., 2011). So it may simply be that depressed people both die earlier and rate their health more pessimistically.

Predictors of age at death are one way of studying health. Another is to study the very old who, by definition, have already exceeded the normal life span and thus may be assumed to harbour a secret of health. Populations containing a high proportion of people living an unusually long time that are currently being studied include Okinawans; Seventh-Day Adventists in Loma Linda, California; and Sardinians.

An important finding from these studies is that long life is associated with having fewer illnesses than the average person. This seems not to be because these are lucky people who have escaped illness, but because being healthy – like having mental well-being – protects against illness. Health protective factors that are consequent on well-being and life satisfaction include a smaller waist and higher dihydroepiandosterone sulfate (a precursor of both male and female sex hormones) in men and lower biochemical markers of inflammation in women, along with lower plasma triglycerides and better lung function in both sexes (Steptoe et al., 2012).

It is likely that genomic markers of health will emerge soon, but two indirect measures that have already been validated are grip strength and telomere length.

Bodily strength is a weak measure of health. Human DNA is not only to be found in the cell nucleus, but in the energy-producing organelles, the mitochondria. These probably have their own DNA because they were once independent organisms that first parasitized vertebrate cells and then became useful partners or symbionts. They are transmitted to the next generation in the cytoplasm of the egg. So we all get our DNA from our mothers, and it may be significant that maternal age at death is a more important predictor of our life expectancy than paternal age. Since mitochondria also produce our energy, they may be linked to the vitality that is associated with increased physical activity and therefore health. Some studies have been conducted on the relevance to life expectancy of having one particular variant of mitochondrial DNA rather than another, and there does appear to be a link (Niemi et al., 2003).

Grip strength is a more specific measure of health. Grip strength, adjusted for body size, predicts all-cause mortality even if measured many years before death (Oksuzyan et al., 2010). Fall in grip strength, which usually occurs after the onset of the 60s, as well as reduced absolute grip strength, is also associated with risk of disability and reduced life expectancy (Starr & Deary, 2011). However, grip strength is not simply a measure of physical endowment. It is also a measure of continued physical activity, which is known to be linked to health (Matthews et al., 2007; Rantanen et al., 2012).

Grip strength is correlated with socioeconomic status as a child (Starr & Deary, 2011). Commonsense psychology has had a weak grip down as a measure of disapproval, perhaps because the handshakes of high status and highly confident individuals are typically firm.

Grip strength may therefore be a particularly good measure of health because it is not purely biological, but also influenced by personal and social factors.

Telomeres are repeats of the nonsense codons TTAGGG (the letters refer to the bases thiamine, adenine and guanine) at the 3' end of each chromosome. In life, the chromosome is folded so that the 3' end doubles back to somewhere close to the anchor point of two paired chromosomes (the centromere) where it is linked to a loop of DNA in the other chromosome in the pair. It is therefore like a kind of popper, although its importance may not be so much structural as acting as a stop signal to RNA transcription (Ly, 2009). Telomere length normally shortens with each cell division and therefore with age. This is not the case with cancer cells, and may be one reason that these cells do not die and that the cancer therefore grows uncontrollably. Starting with longer telomeres appears to be associated with longevity in some organisms (Heidinger et al., 2012) although the jury is out in humans. The rate of shortening does appear to be inversely associated with reduced life expectancy (Nakamura et al., 2007). However, like grip strength, a reduction in telomere length is not purely a matter of intrinsic biology as it is also associated with childhood social status (Cherkas et al., 2006) and even with whether one's mother experiences adverse life events whilst one is still in the womb (Entringer et al., 2011). Telomere length is also affected by adversity after birth. This may account for the increases and decreases in telomere length that occur over quite short periods of time (Svenson et al., 2011).

Adaptation

Psychiatrists and psychologists have tried to grapple with the stigma attached to mental disorders for decades, not least because stigma is, itself, a cause of future breakdown. For a while, it seemed important to do this by using politically correct language. Neuroses were re-termed 'maladaptive responses'. This was shrewd as it focused on the idea that a neurosis was not an abnormal response, but a response that was not going to be fit for purpose. The word 'fit' introduces another word often used in relation to health – 'fitness'. Fitness and adaptation are also words used in evolution theory to capture the idea that a species may survive for a long time not because it is perfectly adapted to its current ecological niche, but because it is not, or, rather, because it has the potential to adapt as its niche changes. This may be for various reasons – the presence of latent genes, the ability to make rapid genetic changes or the durability of a design that survives in many different environments (think of crocodiles or cockroaches).

An alternative definition of health to the WHO one that presupposes a particular state is that based on adaptability (Huber et al., 2011). Health is, according to this definition, a capacity, the capacity to adapt to environmental change without loss of function.

Healthy happiness

We have noted many times already in previous chapters that good health and happiness are inter-correlated (Judge et al., 2010). The way that we think about them is also very similar. We consider that ill health is the inverse of good health, just as unhappiness is the inverse of happiness, but we recognize that what makes a person less unhealthy does not make them healthy, any more than what makes someone less unhappy does not make them happy.

The relationship between unhappiness and ill health is less clear. A recent review of the literature concludes that they are independent of each other (Friedman & Kern, 2013), but this is contrary to several studies which show that feeling negative about life generally increases the risk of developing a physical disorder (Weiser, 2012) and persistent negative feelings increase all-cause mortality (Russ et al., 2012), though not if the downswing is a temporary response to adversity (Ventegodt et al., 2006). The evidence that depression leads to poor health is even stronger.

It was a surprise when community studies of physical symptoms got going, more or less at the same time after the Second World War, how few people considered themselves healthy. Aches and pains are warning signals that stop us over-using our bodies and might be considered to be healthy, but in these studies they were being taken to be indicators of disorder. Only a minority of people with aches and pains, limited mobility, shortness of breath, headaches or other symptoms have a physical disorder that will persist, however, just as only a minority of people who feel stressed, worried or fed up have a persistent mental disorder. The difference is not merely quantitative. In one large US sample, participants rated their emotions and other indices of mental health and well-being. The presence or absence of a disorder – generalized anxiety disorder, major depression, panic disorder and alcohol dependence – and happiness and well-being were correlated, but each made an independent contribution to the participants feeling helpless, close to others, sure of where they were going in life and able to work a full day without taking time off sick (Keyes, 2005).

Happiness can mean just having a happy feeling or it can mean a disposition to having happy feelings. We have mainly used it in this second sense – the sense that Diener has called 'subjective well-being'. A disposition is not purely a reflection of our emotional settings – of our 'hedonic balance' – but incorporates evaluations too. A person who loves the country is, for example, not so disposed to happiness whilst living in the city as someone who loves the bright lights. Happiness is therefore never going to be something that can be measured against an objective and universal scale. Health can be, however, if we accept that years of life (perhaps adjusted for quality of life) are the ability of the body to deal with and survive the challenges that life, and senescence, throws at it.

Centenarians are, on this measure, healthier than the general population because they have outlived the rest of us. Centenarians can be expected to have been happier throughout their lives than their shorter-lived fellow citizens, too, since happiness and health are linked, and indeed a positive attitude to life is a common feature of centenarian populations (Kato et al., 2012). However, a disposition to feeling positive does not itself seem like a survival characteristic, since being positive when in a jam would not seem like the best motivator to do something about it. What might then be of survival value would be some anger to motivate one to confront someone or something blocking one's path, or some anxiety to tune into, and therefore avoid, threats or dangers.

So are there some features of centenarian psychological adjustment that give some clues about the particular kind of happiness that is most healthy? Three consistent features are positive feelings, a lack of negative feelings and conscientiousness (Terracciano et al., 2008). The first two are predictable from the evidence that we have already presented in this chapter, but conscientiousness suggests that we were right in speculating that feeling good is not enough. A happy and healthy life also requires that one has standards and sticks to them even when it is difficult to do so. Health happiness is therefore very close to what we noted in the previous chapter, to what psychologists would call life satisfaction, i.e. a kind of happiness that comes from engagement in life rather than detachment from it.

Factors that influence health

Genetic factors

Genetic factors are increasingly seen as important for health but despite intense research there is no consensus about what these are (Slagboom et al., 2011), although maternal age at death may be a more important determinant than paternal age, pointing to the possible importance of mitochondria in health that we have already mentioned.

Purely genetic research is being replaced by genomic studies, which take account of the interactions between genes and epigenetic influences of the environment and of developmental changes in the expression of the genome. According to this newer view, we are not determined by our genetic endowment, but rather genes provide a horizon in which our actions and our environment influence how our genes are expressed.

Psychosocial factors

Social status and social support are associated with happiness and negatively associated with depression but make independent contributions to longevity.

Social status has been extensively studied in two cohorts of British civil servants (Whitehall Studies I and II) (Marmot, 2004) and found to be continuously correlated with health, such that each incremental rise in social status is associated with an increase in health. The finding has been replicated in other populations, and other countries, and holds whether status is measured or estimated by income, occupational status or education.

Sir Michael Marmot, who led the Whitehall studies, has since created a research group to study the interaction of social and health inequalities, and considers that a likely mediating factor is autonomy or the absence of constraint on a person's plans and intentions. Positive affect in conjunction with autonomy increases people's determination to achieve personal goals (Haase et al., 2012). Self-efficacy, a related concept, also accounts for the links between positive feelings, spirituality and health (Konopack & McAuley, 2012).

Social support is an additional factor in some studies of health, whether directly measured as the number of social contacts one has or indirectly as loneliness. Social support could be related to autonomy, since the ability to mobilize the help of others in plans is an important contributor to autonomy. It could be a buffer against negative feelings but it may also be an index of engagement.

Engagement in life – creativity, social or family involvement – may be another independent health-promoting factor.

Activity and body mass

There is much evidence linking exercise and average body weight with longevity (Berrington de Gonzalez et al., 2010) but, like many other health-related factors, it is not clear what the causal pathway is. Activity and body mass are themselves inter-correlated and both are also linked with chronic medical conditions, including depression, possibly being a cause of these conditions or, alternatively, being a consequence of them (Hawker, 2012). The only way to sort out these factors is through longitudinal studies, and several such studies have begun recently.

Sexual intercourse

Health has complex relationships with sexual intercourse. Increased frequency of intercourse may be associated with multiple partners, which increases the risk of the transmission of sexually transmitted disease, and may also be associated with forced sex in women. Satisfaction with sex in women in stable relationships is correlated with life satisfaction, but this may not hold true for men (Walfisch et al., 1984). No general conclusions can be reached about sexual intercourse and health. There is no support for the commonly held view that men 'need' sexual satisfaction.

Despite this, the frequency or experienced quality of sexual intercourse is often cited as the most important contributor to happiness, and even well-being, especially of men. There have been few empirical studies of the frequency of sexual intercourse and happiness, and none of the intensity of pleasure given by intercourse and happiness, that seems to dominate more popular sexology. Even longitudinal studies cannot deal entirely with the issue of whether happiness means that people have more sex, or vice versa (Wadsworth, 2013). Wadsworth did find a strong positive correlation between the frequency of sexual intercourse and self-rated happiness, but there was a negative correlation of happiness with perceived frequency of intercourse in a reference group. Taking these two findings into account, Wadsworth concluded that having sex more often than the neighbours were perceived to be having it was most strongly associated with happiness.

Smoking

Smoking vegetable products, whether tobacco or cannabis, is associated with poorer health and reduced life expectancy.

Alcohol

Alcohol use is also associated with poorer health and reduced life expectancy, but this may be offset by the beneficial effects of alcohol, if indeed there are any. There is considerable controversy about this, but there is a growing consensus that red wine drinking is associated with increased longevity in some populations.

The link between red wine and long life was disputed by purists who thought of alcohol as being an evil, and hailed by hedonists who wanted it to be the alcohol and not anything specific to red wine itself that was life-enhancing.

The evidence seems to point to there being a particular group of compounds in red wine, of which one of the most important is resveratrol, that do have a health-inducing effect, by stimulating mitochondrial energy production. Resveratrol does this via a gene, SIRT1, that is present in different doses in different people. SIRT1 is involved in a number of processes within the cell, but the relevant one increases the production of mitochondria

(Price et al., 2012). It also plays a role in telomere length. So the benefits of red wine do seem to be real but confined to those people with SIRT1.

Nutrition

Another contentious area is whether there are some diets that are healthier than others. There is general agreement that low levels of saturated fat, high antioxidant intake and low glycemic load are all features of a healthy diet (Willcox et al., 2009), but whether there are specific dietary elements that are protective is open to debate.

So a diet low in animal fats, including dairy products, low in sucrose and high in fruit and vegetables is a good bet. However, native Siberians who do not adopt Western culture have a normal life expectancy, even though their diet mainly consists of animal meat, whereas the Alaskan Yup'ik, who adopt a Westernized lifestyle, have a reduced life expectancy, probably through their excessive use of drink and drugs (Wolsko et al., 2007).

It seems likely that the effects of nutrition, like the effects of wine, vary from individual to individual, depending on the genomic factors determining their metabolism.

Vitality

Minkowski, the psychiatrist not the mathematician, was a Lithuanian who trained in medicine in Poland, in psychiatry in Switzerland and practised in France. He was much influenced by the French philosopher Bergson, and applied Bergson's ideas about time to his practice by distinguishing between his patients who lived in the past, those who lived in the present and those who lived for the future. He also applied Bergson's concept of 'élan vital' to individuals. Bergson's idea was that cultures differed in their vitality. Minkowski thought that individuals, too, had a characteristic 'vitality', which he called 'élan personnel'. Similar ideas were advanced by psychoanalysts in the interwar period. Karl Menninger coined the term 'vital energy' and Gerald Caplan, 'narcissistic supplies', both terms being derived from the hydraulic theory of libido of the early Freud.

These ideas fell out of fashion as psychoanalysis did. They were too tied up, perhaps, with the warrior mentality and inconsistent with the humanistic revolution in health studies, which rejected 'positivism'. However, as we have considered above, some determinants of health do seem to be related to energy production at a cellular level. Positive feelings, too, function as a kind of energy – an energy for engagement, for tackling novelty, for making new relations.

Creativity is another factor independently linked to longevity. Subjective accounts of what creativity adds to life often cite terms like 'zest' or 'passion' that imply increased energy for living.

Victory and defeat

As already noted, Nietzsche wrote, 'what does not kill us makes us strong'. There is some evidence for this. It is how the immune system works, for example. An infection by a potentially lethal organism, if the infection is overcome by the immune system, results in lymphocytes that possess DNA that can quickly synthesize antibodies that will bind with some part of the pathogen, enabling it to be readily eaten and destroyed by macrophages during the early stages of any future re-infection. The same idea is fundamental to several theories of the response to adversity, including stress-inoculation theory, resilience and coping theory. However, in both physical and mental health there are also opposing theories, that some kind of earlier insult, damage or threat may leave a hidden vulnerability, making a person more open to future adversity. Psychoanalysts argue that psychological trauma works like this, for example.

The difference between the two kinds of theory turns on whether the first challenge is victoriously overcome or whether the victory is a Pyrrhic one. A trivial example of this is infection by one of the large herpes viruses. These are viruses that co-exist with the cellular machinery of their host. If chicken pox is completely overcome by the child who gets it, this leads to lifelong immunity. But if the virus lives on in the child's cells despite being cleared from the blood, the child's victory over the virus is partial at best. For later in life, often very late in life, when the immune system is weak or during some kind of adversity, the virus may start to divide again and burst out of its host cells, leading to a limited outbreak of chicken pox or, as it is then called, shingles (herpes zoster).

A person who has survived chicken pox may therefore have been completely victorious over it, in which case their health is enhanced, or they may have been partly, but cryptically, defeated, in which case their health is reduced.

I am here adopting a military metaphor for health, a metaphor that was often used by Freud when considering mental health in terms of 'defences', but an even more influential metaphor for maintaining health comes from mechanical engineering.

Stress

Hans Selye, an endocrinologist, introduced the metaphor 'stress' from engineering to account for animals' reactions to noxious stimuli, including inoculations (Selye, 1998). He found that there was increased activity in two juxtaposed tissues, the adrenal medulla and the adrenal cortex, in response to any challenge that threatened the animal's survival. The initial response was an increase in the size and activity of the tissues of the inner, medullary, part of the adrenal gland, the organ concerned with, as we now know, increased production of epinephrine and norepinephrine. But in the longer run, it was the outer, cortical, part of the gland that showed the greatest increase in size, a part associated with an increase in the secretion in the cortex of the eponymously named steroid hormones or corticosteroids like cortisol (leaving out the other steroids produced in the adrenal cortex such as the mineralocorticoids and the sex hormones). Brain structures controlling the gland, the pituitary (and we now know, the hypothalamus in the base of the brain) were noticed by Selye to be enlarged too.

Enlargement and evidence of increased secretion was the first reaction to stress, which Selye (1998) termed the 'general alarm reaction'. The enlarged organs were able to produce the raised amounts of hormone required to deal with prolonged stress and this Selye called the 'general adaptation syndrome'. However, there was a limit to enlargement and to secretory capacity and then the third phase of stress set in – 'exhaustion'. Exhaustion is a physical health state but it often coincides with a psychological experience of 'defeat' (Gilbert & Allan, 1998), to revert to our military metaphor.

The relationship between bodily reactions and emotions is not as simple as it seemed to scientists like Selye in the 1930s. Steroid depletion (Selye's exhaustion phase) can be reversed by giving injections of cortisol, but emotional defeat cannot be reversed by a physical intervention. When someone says that they are 'stressed', they are making no comment about their own emotional reactions to this outside force, and this may correspond to the phase of adaptation, when there is increased arousal, as well as to the stage of exhaustion, when arousal flags.

There is an assumption, too, that everyone gets stressed by the same things and in the same way. This is useful in ordinary conversation as no one, neither the speaker nor the casual listener, wants to engage enough with another to know exactly what negative feelings they have and why they have them. However, what stresses one person does not stress another and when one person gets anxious, another person drinks or gives up. But all of them may attribute this to stress. Difficulty, pressure and hard work are not in themselves causes of stress or ill health (Friedman & Kern, 2013).

The importance of Selye's model is that it accounts both for what I call victory over adversity and defeat. When people describe feeling stressed, what they mean is that they are beginning to feel defeated by some stressor, whether that is a demand for work success that they cannot meet, a relationship conflict that they cannot sort out or some kind of unremitting trauma or adversity. The importance of feeling stressed is that our concern switches away from achieving our aims in life to focusing down on relieving the stress, and it is at this point that we start to feel ill.

Ill health and unhappiness

Illness, in our definition, is when our health is defeated by the demands placed on it. We do not need to have a definition of health to know this moment: it is when our purposes shrink down to looking after ourselves or being looked after, as Aristotle noted in the *Nicomachean Ethics*. Other kinds of adversity can also shrink our horizons in this way. Aristotle mentions the man short of money, who can only think of how to find the price of a meal or lodging. Thirst, hunger, fear of attack – all of these can make living the good life take second place to finding the means to survive.

When our health fails, our conception of well-being changes. We cease to take well-being for granted as a by-product of living well, and start to see it as a good, or even as a property, which is ours by right. We want it to be given back. We become selfish about it, if necessary paying through the nose for remedies and, if necessary, outbidding others to get them.

This may be one explanation for the massive spending in the Western world on health care (really illness care), compared to the much smaller amount spent on health promotion and preventative medicine. It may also explain the high status accorded to doctors who, of all health professionals, have the most effective remedies for illness available.

This high status may also explain the contempt that is sometimes shown for the 'medical model' that sees health merely as the absence of illness. Medical investigation has only touched on the detection of health, as we saw above, and not at all on the detection of happiness, but has a considerable range of methods to detect illness and even some to detect unhappiness and anxiety.

Doctors' relative disinterest in positive health is understandable, given that most of their patients are only concerned about their health when they are ill, but this has had an alarming effect.

Medicalization of the body and mind

Suppose one of us is unhappy. What do we do? Do we think that we need to grin and bear it? Do we think that we are depressed and need something to relieve it – a holiday perhaps or a course of therapy? Or do we ask ourselves what am I unhappy about, on the assumption that there must be something? The first two reactions are based on the medical model. The last is based on a quite different approach that I will call 'existential'. There is no best or right evaluation. Sometimes emotions do come and go, and we can afford to ignore them. At other times, people get depressed for purely physical reasons: in bipolar disorder, for example, or after childbirth, or in response to certain drugs given for other conditions. However, critics of the medical model argue that accidental causes of poor health are much rarer than doctors would have us believe. It is more that doctors have a restless need to fix things that drugs or other interventions are prescribed, rather than the reasons for poor health being looked into. The critics go on to say that the offer of quick fixes for poor health or unhappiness chimes with a child-like wish on all our parts that someone will fix us up when things go wrong. Medicine tends to aggravate the desire to be fixed. Doctors and pharmaceutical researchers value success in fixing so many diseases encourage patients to accept that low mood is a problem to be fixed and not a signal of something that needs attention.

Let's take an example. We are woken by chest pain at night and recognize that it is indigestion. Do we go to a doctor asking for confirmation that we have gastric reflux, in which case we are likely to be prescribed a proton pump inhibitor, or do we ask whether we are eating a diet that is right for us? Some people do have an incompetent cardiac sphincter and are pathologically prone to reflux, but many of them would have a more fully functioning sphincter if they lost weight.

Preventative medicine

Doctors in some states are willing to be the servants of the state. Some doctors are willing to give lethal injections, to supervise judicial amputations, to supervise the insertion of stomach tubes into prisoners on hunger strike, and so on. All of these activities are clearly not in the interests of the recipients of medical attention and are therefore violations of medical ethics. Many formulations of medical ethics begin with the notion of a contract between the doctor and the patient that takes priority over any contract that the doctor might have with a third party. But in all parts of the world, and every day, doctors breach this principle by acting on unconscious patients, assuming that they know what is in those patients' best interests, and compulsorily treating unwilling patients who present a danger through violence associated with medical illness or because of a physical illness that can be spread to other people.

Conservative groups of doctors, such as members of the American Medical Association, are so unwilling to find themselves in this position that they have consistently blocked efforts to introduce 'third-party payers', such as insurance companies or state reimbursement schemes, and are adamantly opposed to schemes like the British NHS where doctors are directly employed by government or, rather, government-sponsored proxies, currently called NHS trusts.

Employed doctors do not however need to treat as many individual patients as possible to maintain their income, leaving them time to treat communities as well. Arguably, it is this kind of health care, 'public health', that has had the biggest impact on illness through the implementation of preventative measures against the big killers of the past: industrial injuries, road traffic accidents, infections and environmental toxins.

Many doctors now consider that there are new medical hazards on the horizon which preventative medicine should address. These include poverty, inequality (a goal championed by two medical knights, Douglas Black and Michael Marmot), nuclear war, bad teeth, goitre, excessive fat, salt and sugar ingestion, physical chastisement, exposure to violence in the workplace, long hours of work, being thrown through the windscreens of our cars and over-use of antibiotics.

In the UK, legislation exists to insist that people wear seatbelts, water companies fluoridate water, salt manufacturers put iodide into flour, and so on. But these are all examples of governments exercising parental or 'nanny' rights over their citizens. There are those in the USA who consider that this contravenes the US Declaration of Independence that states that it is a self-evident truth that everyone is endowed with 'certain unalienable Rights, that among these are Life, Liberty and the pursuit of Happiness' (Gwinnett, 1776). It follows that everyone has the right not to be obstructed in their pursuit of happiness, but not that everyone has a right to happiness. It also implies that if a person pursues happiness at the expense of their health, then they should be at liberty to do so.

The founding fathers of the United States were thinking of King George of England and his governors, and their imposition of taxes and other restrictions, which stopped the colonists from being happy. But the suspicions of George III have carried over to suspicions of any central authority imposing itself on the individual citizen. This may be one explanation for why more is spent on health care on average by each US citizen than is spent anywhere else in the world, and yet the mortality rate in the USA, and thereby US health, is well below that of many other countries.

Dealing with illness

Sooner or later, everyone gets ill. The most serious illnesses, or at least those requiring the most expensive care, typically occur in the last five years of life. In fact, the onset of a succession of life-threatening illnesses, even if they can be treated effectively, is an indicator that the last five years have been reached.

'Symptoms' and 'signs' are the basis of the medical viewpoint. Symptoms intrude into consciousness as warnings of some malfunction. They may be bodily symptoms, in which case they are alerting us to our bodies. Or they may be mental symptoms, in which case they are telling us about our minds or about our social situation. Signs are indications of malfunction that other people observe. This may be by direct observation – for example, the swelling in the neck or 'goitre' of someone with thyroid disease – or as a result of special tests – for example, the white spot on the CT scan of someone with a tumour.

For simplicity, we shall use the term 'symptoms' to include signs in the remainder of this chapter.

The appearance of a new symptom of illness creates a kind of challenge which might not at this initial stage be too threatening. People have symptoms of some kind a lot, and one of the functions of experts is to reassure them that they are harmless, as much of the time they indeed are (Diener et al., 1999). If they are not harmless, then the symptom becomes a threat and a source of worry as well as a stimulus to action. The restoration of health becomes a priority. How well people access effective health care may be influenced by their status and education, as indeed by how quickly they recognize a symptom and how accurately they weigh up the challenge that it poses. There is a considerable literature on each of these steps that I will not summarize. Instead, we will consider the more general theme of overcoming, or being defeated by, illness or indeed any other adversity.

Why do people live longer?

People in developed countries live longer – and are therefore healthier – now than ever before and, so far as is known, can also expect a longer life than any other group in history. The fall in infant mortality has had a disproportionate effect on life expectancy, but the life expectancy of 50-year-olds has also increased. It has been estimated that life expectancy is currently increasing in the West by six hours a day (Blagosklonny, 2010). Life expectancy may be exactly that: how much life we expect to have. People who feel that they are getting old may die young (Hsu et al., 2010). Happiness, as we have noted already, is associated with longevity as is status. These effects may be independent of intervening variables such as diet or access to preventive medical interventions such as vaccination (Cherkas et al., 2006). Extreme physical labour, often linked to status, may shorten life, as may extreme inactivity. Both may be linked to low mood. Servitude, slavery or labour exploitation shorten life, as Marx and Engels noted (Marx, 1961).

Clean water, sewage disposal, fresh food, safer environments and protection from attack by vigilantes, brigands and armies have been some of the health measures instituted by governments, often acting on the advice of public health officials who have monitored birth and death statistics. So changes at the public level as well as at the private level have also played a part.

Less and less people consider themselves to be the slave of another person. The machine revolution that has rendered us more immobile has also made us much less dependent on the mindless labour of other human beings. More and more people therefore consider that they can claim a full set of human rights. In turn they impose a full set of duties on the states in which they live. So the improvement in personal health and in the public health may be linked. Autonomy, it has been argued by Sir Michael Marmot (Marmot, 2004), is the mediating factor between employment status and health. As noted in a previous chapter, many of us now aspire to the same autonomy as would have been granted only to warriors or private gentlemen in the societies of Northern Greece, the Indus or the Yangtse valleys in the late Bronze Age, around the 5th century BCE; and many of us are able to achieve it. It is not therefore surprising that there is a general interest in the philosophers who emerged around this time: they include the ancient Greek philosophers that we considered in Chapter 1, the anonymous authors of the Vedas and the Mahabharata, and the posthumously recorded writings of Master Kong in China.

These philosophies were written for those people who not only led in their community in peace time but in war. In the Indus valley, they emerged as a specific class, the Ksatriya, which was distinct from the hereditary caste of the priests. They took exploitation of other human beings for granted, along with the legitimacy of violence as a tool of government.

In the contemporary world, these warrior values have not disappeared but are no longer considered unproblematic. Murder, assassination, warfare, enslavement, domestic violence, childhood sexual and physical abuse – these are all bad for the health as well as being morally bad. We will consider in the next chapter whether they might also be bad for the well-being of the perpetrator.

Defeat, unhappiness and ill health

Seligman, the influential founder of positive psychology, had begun his psychological research with a study of learned helplessness (Seligman, 1975). One model of this was to make rats jump from electrified platforms to other, non-electrified ones. Rats showed an aversion to standing on a platform that had been electrified even if it was no longer carrying current, and so they jumped off. However, if the experimenter began to electrify the platform that they were jumping to, so that the rats had nowhere to jump safely, they stopped jumping away from the platform but instead stood there, shivering and looking as if they were paralysed by fear. These rats pined, went off their food and died prematurely. Seligman called the state that the rats were in 'learned helplessness', but it has clear affinities with the state that Selye (1998) called 'exhaustion'. Seligman thought that learned helplessness was a model for depression, giving the example of his own father, a miner, who had been made redundant during a mining downturn and had pined away and died.

Lester Luborsky once undertook an intensive study of those of his patients in long-term psychoanalytic psychotherapy who also had persistent ill health. He examined the content of sessions before a session in which a patient had reported a worsening of their low mood, phobia, chest pain or missed cardiac beats and he compared it with the content of sessions before an otherwise comparable session in which they reported that their health problems had not been in evidence. In the sessions when patients were going through a phase of symptom recurrence, they spoke more about feeling hopeless, out of control, helpless and lacking support from others: defeated, in other words.

Defeat and illness go together, and this has received further support from studies of immune suppression following adversity (Diener & Chan, 2011). At a trivial level, we know this because we are more likely to succumb to a virus – catch a cold, say – when we are feeling over-tired or overstressed.

Contact with other people may sometimes mitigate the effects of adversity, partly via a direct effect on the immune system (Leserman et al., 2000), and the effect also works in rats (Ruis et al., 1999). One of the reasons that Seligman's rats proved so susceptible to learned helplessness may have been that they were not housed with rats that they knew could offer the post-traumatic grooming that mitigates stress in a rat. Another problem, of course, is that the rats had absolutely no control over what happened to them and, as we saw previously, a lack of autonomy has been linked to ill health in human studies as well.

In fact, it is often difficult to separate out a lack of autonomy, having nowhere to turn, a lack of understanding from others and a feeling that one has run out of energy and ideas oneself. All of these factors together lead to a sense that there is no way forward, only back, and it is a short step from retreat to defeat.

Turning defeat around

Janoff-Bulman argued that a trauma may be so devastating and yet so unwarranted that it strips away what she calls 'the belief in a just world' (Janoff-Bulman, 1992). This kind of defeat cannot easily be challenged because no reliance can ever again be placed on things going right – we will come back to this when we consider the psychotherapist's viewpoint in Chapter 8. Feeling that the adversity is meaningless increases the sense of defeat (Murphy & Johnson, 2003).

Another, or perhaps related, reason for defeats to be irrecoverable is that a person's beliefs about themselves rest on the foundation that they can cope with anything that life throws at them.

There exist many aphorisms that suggest ways we can preserve our amour propre but still accept a temporary defeat – 'I might have lost this battle, but I can still win the war' is one example. The capacity to overcome temporary defeat is often called resilience. Resilience has cognitive elements, such as the coping skills that we considered in the last chapter, and emotional elements. A positive hedonic balance is one emotional factor that results in mood swinging back to the positive even after it has been pushed very strongly into the negative by a loss or a threat. A strong spiritual belief is another factor that increases resilience and we shall consider this in the next chapter.

Defeat and comfort

Some people cope with defeat by believing that they need or deserve comforting by others. Of course, this is often the case in the short term, but in the long term comfort prolongs defeat, just as reassurance prolongs anxiety-proneness. Comfort-related behaviours are often unhealthy. Examples include drinking or smoking more, eating more sweet things, reducing activity and engagement to avoid conflict and depending on medication or drugs for relief. Older people who feel defeated die younger (Fry & Debats, 2011). Defeated anger or shameful defeat may be particularly likely to lead to unhealthy behaviour (Leith & Baumeister, 1996).

Chronic depression and panic disorder are markers of chronic defeat (Gilbert et al., 2002) and are themselves linked to poor health and decreased life expectancy, especially in women (Reynolds et al., 2008). How these effects are mediated is not known but one possible route may be through lifestyle changes, resulting in weight gain.

Is physical disease always defeating?

Many of the physical illnesses that doctors deal with are fatal. Others, even if they are not fatal, are disabling – osteo- and rheumatoid arthritis are examples. Others, even if not disabling through their effects on the musculoskeletal system, may be chronically painful. The question therefore arises, 'Is it possible to have happiness and yet be physically ill?' The answer seems to be that it is, so long as one is not depressed or in chronic pain, and so long as one is not disabled from undertaking activities that are perceived as essential for well-being.

Last thoughts

It will, we hope, have been clear in this chapter that good health and happiness are bound together in positive well-being, but that it is still possible to be happy and in poor health. What might have been less expected by the reader is that it is not possible to be chronically unhappy and in good health. Despite many health warnings (Bonneux et al., 1998), government experts argue that disproportionately too much money is being spent on physical health rather than mental health (Hawkes, 2012) in the UK. There is considerable tolerance for mentally ill people in the abstract in the UK, but 1 in 8 still think that 'one of the main causes of mental illness is a lack of self-discipline and will power' and 1 in 4 think that enough is being spent on the care of people with mental illness already (Health and Social Care Information Centre, 2011).

In this chapter, I have argued that each of us have some responsibility for our own well-being. Failing to exercise it does not mean that we lack discipline or will power. Attributions like this justify a moralistic and rejecting response to the needs of the mentally ill. Better models of akrasia are needed that do not take away responsibility but do not apportion blame, and therefore punishment, either. Social sanctions may just make the situation worse (Dickerson et al., 2004).

5

The Politician's Viewpoint

Relief of poverty is a duty in many religions. It was institutionalized in the UK in 1601 by the Poor Law, which required parishes to succour the poor of the parish. In the late 18th century, Parisian officials considered that poor people flooding into Paris were bringing in disease and created hostels to quarantine them. In the 19th century, a lack of able-bodied soldiers became a concern to officials recruiting an expeditionary force to fight the Boer war. By the end of the 20th century, a widespread welfare policy that had resulted from the government's recognition that it was in the state's interest to look after the poor, and not just a religious duty, had created a new problem, which was that unemployment had both indirect (lost production) and direct costs to the state, but that employment required that workers had the skills and stamina to work with the machines that had become ubiquitous in the workplace.

Most countries have responded to these challenges by considering that well-being and not just health should be a priority target for government. In the UK, a future scoping 'Foresight' programme was designed to interpret and extrapolate the findings of current science into the future, including a thread on 'Mental capital and mental well-being'. The findings were published in *Nature* (Beddington et al., 2008). The authors defined 'mental well-being' from a state's point of view as 'individuals' ability to develop their potential, work productively and creatively, build strong and positive relationships with others and contribute to their community' (2008: 1057).

The Foresight report led to the first UK well-being survey, which has become incorporated as a module of the Opinions and Lifestyle survey carried out monthly in a stratified sample of UK households receiving less than 500 items of post per day. In the first survey, 18,000 UK citizens were asked four questions (see Box 5.1) and the results were collated with the results of other UK surveys.

BOX 5.1   QUESTIONS ASKED IN THE UK OFFICE OF NATIONAL STATISTICS MEASURING NATIONAL WELL-BEING PROGRAMME

1   Overall, how satisfied are you with your life nowadays?
2   Overall, to what extent do you feel the things you do in your life are worthwhile?
3   Overall, how happy do you feel?

Some of the key points were that relationships were an important element in well-being, but 14% of respondents described themselves as being dissatisfied with their social relationships; contact with friends fell curvilinearly with increasing age; and marital satisfaction fell with the length of marriage. Although this might suggest a bleak picture for older people, a third of people with low life satisfaction had low satisfaction with relationships, whilst high life satisfaction was associated in nearly 90% with high relationship satisfaction. This may suggest that respondents who are happy are more likely to attract and engage other people in high quality relationships.

Clearly, this might have implications for government policy. For example, rather than increasing opportunities for older people to interact (less than 10% of the sample went to social groups organized for older people), it would be better to focus on those with persistent negative feelings, who are the least likely to be outgoing and rewarding to be with, a suggestion also made by Lord Layard, as we saw in Chapter 2.

Doing well as a country

What will UK government ministers do with these figures? To give them their due, they have launched a programme to reduce loneliness in older people though without funding it. Politicians are always suspected by those they rule of simply being there for their own advantage, although there is much less basis for this suspicion than in states where corruption and the misuse of power are at much higher levels. But it is true that government priorities are often different to those of the individual voter, often giving rise to the ordinary man in the street's idea that no one in government 'gives a toss' about them.

National security and wealth creation have been two of the main preoccupations of rulers throughout history, and the effective pursuit of these has required attention to the well-being of the general population, but individuals have not always experienced the advantages of these in the way that government expected.

National security

General conscription, introduced in Victorian England to recruit for the Boer war, led to large numbers of young men being medically examined for the first time. The discovery that many of these men were unfit to fight led to the welfare reforms of the early 20th century brought in by Liberal governments. These reforms have probably made a substantial contribution to increased longevity in the UK at the early part of the century, although they were soon implemented by countries not all of whom were intending to fight wars, and the UK's life expectancy is nowadays in the middle of the national league tables for life expectancy.

Wars are often justified on the basis of national security, even if they are apparently offensive. The current war in Afghanistan has been said to be a war on the drugs that are believed to be harming young Westerners. Going to war increases the anxiety of the general population and substantially increases depression and anxiety in combatants and their families. War has a negative effect on well-being and that a government that initiates a war, even if a defensive one, has a responsibility to consider this. Article 35 of the Charter of Fundamental Rights of the European Union states that 'Everyone has the right of access to preventive health care and the right to benefit from medical treatment under the conditions established by national laws and practices. A high level of human health protection shall be ensured in the definition and implementation of all Union policies and activities'. So it is arguable that a government that goes to war is abrogating its duty to provide a high level of human health protection, not just to try and avoid injuries to individual combatants, who might have effectively waived their right to protection under this article, but for their families and neighbours and indeed for a much wider group of people who might be made insecure by news coverage that is threatening.

The long-term consequences of war for the combatants who survive seem to vary with the level of emotional commitment to the aims of the war. The North Vietnamese who participated in the war against South Vietnam do not have worse well-being than non-combatants (Teerawichitchainan & Korinek, 2012) but US combatants in the same war do. A confounding factor here is that there must have been few in North Vietnam who escaped the effects of the war whilst most Americans were insulated from it.

Emotional insecurity is only one side of the insecurity produced by wars. A much greater impact worldwide is the food insecurity that accompanies wars and leads to starvation. Mengistu Haile Mariam was found guilty in absentia of genocide by an Ethiopian court not because he had ordered or been complicit in the murder of many of the opponents of his Derg party, which he had, but because he had ordered large numbers of Ethiopians to move from their traditional farmlands to new settlements, sometimes at the other end of the country, under his 'villagization' policy. This led to widespread starvation but also to hidden human misery. I saw the consequences of this directly in the outpatient clinic of Amanuel Hospital, Addis Ababa, where almost every patient attributed their psychiatric disorder, often anxiety or depression, to this forced migration. The civil war that began at this time and led eventually to the independence of Eritrea was associated with worsening health in children caught up in the conflict (Akresh et al., 2012).

Food insecurity may also be linked to domestic violence and may amplify the effects of the insecurity caused by threat (Chilton & Booth, 2007). Job insecurity is another factor that may contribute to individual insecurity (Ng et al., 2011) and may be a direct consequence of national policies that are, as we see below, aimed at an increase in national wealth.

Wealth and welfare

As soon as rulers are sufficiently wealthy and sufficiently concerned about being toppled by those they rule, they employ advisers to protect them. These advisers may be more in touch with the welfare of individuals in the population. Aristotle and Master Kong were both employed as advisers to kings and both wrote about individual welfare. Welfare was a growing preoccupation of many of the well off in Victorian times with the time and leisure to become politically engaged. Bentham and Mill are good examples.

In the 20th century in the UK, the post-war surge of gratitude to those who had suffered during the course of the war led to the creation of the welfare system and the National Health Service. However, rebuilding the damaged housing stock throughout Europe meant full employment and increased investment did not lead to lay-offs. The gross national product became the index of whether a government was doing well. In the UK, prime minister Harold Macmillan's boast in a speech in 1957 that 'Most of our people have never had it so good' was the prelude to a landslide Tory victory in 1959. But four years later, the downside emerged. The wealth accumulation of the 'get rich quick' generation had outpaced the development of values that would have bridled their greed and concupiscence. Sex scandals in the Tory party emerged. Macmillan resigned, ostensibly on health grounds although he was to live another 23 years. His own personal unhappiness began to emerge. He began to express his survivor guilt. Of the 28 young men who went up to Balliol in 1912, only Macmillan and one other survived the First World War.

Governments began to recognize that their popularity had to rest on a broader base. Some of them turned back to Aristotle.

Robert F. Kennedy, US Attorney General, architect of his brother's successful campaign for US president and later a presidential candidate himself, studied government at Harvard and would, no doubt, have come across Aristotle's *Politics* there. He is reported to have used a quote from Aristotle (possibly a fabricated one) in speeches supporting a reform in health care. In another speech, designed for the children of the newly wealthy at the University of Kansas on 14 March 1968, he listed a series of virtues that made life worthwhile, none of which were being addressed by the focus on wealth:

> Yet the gross national product does not allow for the health of our children, the quality of their education, or the joy of their play. It does not include the beauty of our poetry or the strength of our marriages; the intelligence of our public debate or the integrity of our public officials. It measures neither our wit nor our courage; neither our wisdom nor our learning; neither our compassion nor our devotion to our country; it measures everything, in short, except that which makes life worthwhile. (Rogers, 2012)

Kennedy's sentiments have proved hard to implement in policy. Growth in wealth, many financial experts are convinced, does not lead to well-being in developed societies (Turner, 2010). But the 2012 US presidential campaign was partly fought over whether or not the average American family was worse off than the average Canadian family. As we described in Chapter 2, above a certain level of income, well-being is not correlated with absolute income but with the gap between your income and the income of the person that you compare yourself with. Shifting the comparison to Canada focuses on the rate of growth of the two national economies and is likely to worsen the well-being of voters to the detriment of the incumbent president.

Politicians in developed countries have, we assume, been advised by economists that economic growth cannot continue unabated. For one thing, there is a limit to the natural resources that can fuel expansion. For another, developed countries do not have large, needy populations that provide a reliable market for expanded production. Hence, many politicians have been trying to shift the emphasis from growth in production to an increase in well-being. Robert Kennedy was prescient. Measures of well-being have proliferated. No country has gone so far down this path as Bhutan, and we will consider Bhutan's experience in the next section.

Measuring national well-being

A government intending to replace GDP with a measure of national well-being has the challenge of finding one that will be generally accepted by its citizens. Individual countries, like the UK, are moving towards directly measuring well-being now that GNP is no longer a satisfactory policy target on its own. The worldwide Organisation for Economic Co-operation and Development (OECD) is developing guidelines to assist them with measures of life satisfaction, positive feelings, negative feelings and purpose and meaning of life. These will be applied in a number of different domains.

However, the measurement is likely to become complex and may turn out to be hard to interpret, judging from the experience of one country, Bhutan, which introduced a Gross National Happiness Index to replace their GNP.

The concept of a Gross National Happiness Index was devised by the fourth king of Bhutan, Jigme Singye Wangchuck, in 1974 and was to replace the GNP as the objective of good governance in Bhutan. Article 9, 'the state shall strive to promote those conditions that will enable the pursuit of Gross National Happiness', was added to the constitution and an index of Gross National Happiness was devised (Tobgay et al., 2011). The index was based on the kind of research that we have been reviewing in this book, but also on the government's ideas about what they wanted for the future of Bhutan, with particular emphasis being given to Buddhist values.

The index raises several issues for other governments. The first is that its 33 indicators do not seem able to predict those people who are highly satisfied with their lives. In a report on the 2010 survey using the index, the authors (Ura et al., 2012) give illustrations of four deeply happy people, but each of them has a different indicator profile. A married corporate employee aged 35 living in a town said that his happiness was due to his good health, his basic needs being met, being religious and having peace in the family. A married woman aged 44 runs a farm in the country. She is illiterate, is bothered by animals eating her crop and never forgives, but she is very satisfied with her life, and puts this down to household work, enjoying lifting potatoes and weaving. A 70-year-old widowed monk living in the country has no formal education, sleeps less than most (probably because he meditates a lot), has poor housing and does not know much about the government. He is highly satisfied with life because he can get food from the land. The final example of high satisfaction quoted by Ura et al. (2012) is an unmarried 26-year-old civil servant living alone in a town. She feels that she does not belong but attributes her life satisfaction to love, family, friends, education and having enough money.

It might be difficult, if these examples are anything to go by, for the Bhutanese government to identify obstacles to their citizens' pursuit of happiness that apply to all or even most. A further difficulty is that the government clearly has its own agenda. Indicators include good manners, knowledge of traditional crafts and participation in Buddhist festivals, all valued activities held by the government or its advisers but not necessarily by the Bhutanese themselves. Less than 60% of respondents were, for example, considered 'sufficient' in *Driglam Namzha* or good manners.

Social capital

It might be supposed that, given such a range of differences between citizens' bases for life satisfaction, governments should not concern themselves with promoting happiness, but focus rather, as the Bhutan constitution echoes the Declaration of Independence in saying, on removing obstacles to the pursuit of happiness. However, both well-being and life satisfaction are influenced by others. There are the obvious ways, for example the spread of disease, which affects the health of others, but there are indirect ways as well. For example, more people play tennis during Wimbledon fortnight than at any other time in the UK because they are emulating the players that they see on television. These social influences on well-being and life satisfaction are often considered by economists, who accordingly call them 'social capital'.

The origins of social capital go back to Durkheim (1984), who described 'solidarity' within society which might either be 'mechanical' – solidarity with like-minded fellows in similar walks of life, sometimes called 'bonding capital' – or organic – solidarity with people on whom one is economically interdependent but who are in different walks of life, and sometimes called 'bridging capital' (Putnam, 2000). The term 'social capital' was developed by Pierre Bourdieu (1986) who thought of it as the resources that the people in one's social network could provide. He also posited a cultural capital.

Bridging capital is enhanced by fostering amicable community relations between groups with different values. Bonding capital is most evident in family groups who remain geographically close, and have frequent contact, although as most social contact now takes place on the internet, geographical proximity is less important than shared interests or concerns (Drentea & Moren-Cross, 2005). Measures of social capital have included social participation, contact with friends, perceptions of crime, neighbourhood attachment, social support and self-reports of health and emotional disorder (Pevalin & Rose, 2003). Mostly, we are unaware of social capital since its effects are largely on our mood – what Heidegger called our emotional weather. One study has suggested that we catch happiness or unhappiness from our friends. Another study held that church-going in our neighbourhood enhances our life satisfaction, even if we are not believers ourselves. A third is that the number of broken windows in a neighbourhood is linked to racial prejudice. Social capital applies to health as well as to well-being. A high level of disability or poor health in an important reference group reduces our self-rated health (Carrieri, 2012).

Values

Individuals are more satisfied with life if they are prospering in the areas of life that they most value, and are similarly more dissatisfied if a valued goal or wish is frustrated than if they fail in some goal or desire that they consider of little value. Clearly, the four individuals cited by Ura et al. (2012) had very different values. Governments, too, have values that they often list in a manifesto, and when their values clash with those of individuals, the latter will feel that some of their life satisfaction has been diminished. Politicians hope that their values will match most of the electorate because that will get them re-elected, but they also have their own values, the values of their party and other groups to which they belong, and values that inhere in the parens patriae principle. Politicians, especially powerful ones, often come to believe that they are the parent of their fellow citizens. Parents sometimes believe that they must teach or even impose their values on their children, and politicians sometimes believe the same.

Value conflicts between state and individual can substantially reduce the individual's quality of life, and if the individual fights back, that leads to insecurity within the state, creating fear and other negative feelings in other individuals. However, there are occasions when politicians do lead beneficial national changes that are later adopted by individuals. Modern examples might be the abolition of laws against suicide and homosexual acts in many countries, and the introduction of laws against smoking in public buildings, against racist or sexist behaviour, against cruelty to animals and permitting the termination of pregnancy under certain defined circumstances. Although this list seems rather random, each of these initiatives by legislators was opposed by at least one vociferous group who argued that their fundamental freedoms were being imperilled, or that values vital to the continuance of civilized society were under attack, or both.

Politics and values

The Bhutan surveys cited above show that values are important to well-being. Some of the most influential values are under partial political control, the most conspicuous being corruption and oppression. Corruption at its most mundane is an easy way for politicians to minimize the wage costs of public employees. Pay doctors, customs officers, police officers or civil servants next to nothing and the public will quickly find that they can gain preferential treatment by giving a bribe. This soon becomes routine, such that people who do not give, or cannot afford, a bribe are ill-treated. Corruption widens inequality not just of wealth but of influence. People who know people can use that knowledge to get preferential treatment in a corrupt society.

Corrupt government decreases well-being in citizens (Tavits, 2008), so stamping out corrupt governance is a measure that any government can take to increase national well-being. However, it may not be so easy to do this, not because the average citizen would object but because many of those in power have come to consider bribes, scams and rake-offs as their due.

Oppression is another governmental characteristic that might seem easy to outlaw as it is rarely desired by those who experience it. Oppression may seem justifiable to those who practise it, either because the oppressed are different from other members of the population and are deserving of ill-treatment, the oppression is a kind of discipline to suppress the unruly or the oppression of a particular group prevents that group from becoming a danger to the state or to its officers and servants. In the latter situation, the government might consider house arrest or preventative detention as being fully justified whilst the victims might consider it oppression. Oppression might be much more extreme, running from state-sponsored violence towards dissidents to state employees targeting street children, people with mental illness and people of particular ethnicities for beatings or murder. The development of the first international code of human rights was a response to the Holocaust, which began with the murder of German citizens by the German government. Since then, codes and conventions on human rights have been one of the principal ways to reduce state oppression and, as a result, governmental respect for human rights is linked to an increase in the well-being of those being governed (Talbott, 2010).

It has been argued that justice, and living in a just society, may be an underlying common factor in other political values (Prilleltensky, 2012).

What can improve national well-being?

The recently published 'World Happiness Report' (Helliwell et al., 2012) refers to three international surveys of happiness, but there are many more. Mostly, their results converge on the same league table of happiness, headed usually by Scandinavian countries. Some of the results are hard to believe: for example, that Somalian residents have some of the lowest scores of negative feelings in the world (perhaps living in a failed state is not as bad as people make out).

But the report goes on to consider what governments should take into account when acting to improve their well-being (actually the term that is used is 'happiness' but its use is closer to our use of well-being so we use well-being instead). Layard et al. (2012), in Chapter 3 of the report, consider that there are eight important domains of influence on well-being (see Box 5.2) – four external (likely to be mainly of interest to government) and four personal.

BOX 5.2   DETERMINANTS OF NATIONAL WELL-BEING FROM LAYARD ET AL. (2012)

External:

- income
- work
- community and governance
- values and religion.

Personal:

- mental and physical health
- family experience
- education
- gender and age.

We have already considered many of these and will consider values and religion along with work as a creative enterprise in Chapter 7, and family experience in Chapter 8.

Layard et al. (2012) go on to use econometrics to estimate what proportion of well-being can be attributed to each domain. One important factor that they note is that all of the factors that affect well-being also affect each other. So they use statistical methods (principally analysis of variance) to disentangle them. Income is particularly linked to other factors, for obvious reasons. For example, a higher level of education typically leads to a higher income during working life, and so the two are correlated. When this correlation is allowed for, education makes depressingly little difference to well-being (Oreopoulos & Salvanes, 2011). The school teacher's hope that she or he will be opening children's eyes and ears to the rewarding world of culture may be a delusion.

Employment is also linked to income, but work may be more or less satisfying or more or less threatening too, and the loss of employment may be positive, for example on retirement, or negative, for example on being made redundant.

Layard et al. (2012) conclude that depression and anxiety (or at least what they call malaise) is one of the three most important determinants of future happiness. Using data from the British Cohort Study (Economic and Social Data Service, 2012), they calculate that 10% of the variance in well-being is accounted for by income, 10% by physical health status eight years previously and 23% by depression or anxiety ('malaise') eight years previously. The rest of the variance is accounted for by many other factors, each of which have a much smaller effect, or a large effect only in a minority of people.

Layard et al. suggest that the UK government would be advised to focus on mental health care for older people, following the publication of the first wave of ONS resu

:ll-being programme, and indeed successive UK governments have been persuaded to increase services for people with depression and anxiety by creating a new service, the Improving Access to Psychological Treatment (IAPT) service.

Arguments for the IAPT service were not primarily about promoting well-being but about reducing government expenditure by reducing welfare spending and therefore taxation. There was no appeal to economic growth. Politicians had, it seemed, accepted two main conclusions of the Layard report, that:

1. In a typical country, economic growth improves happiness, other things being equal. But other things are not necessarily equal, so economic growth does not automatically go with increased happiness. Thus policy-makers should balance the argument for more rapid growth against the arguments for supporting other sources of happiness. This applies to countries at every level of development.

2. In developed countries in particular, there is strong micro-level evidence of the importance of income comparisons, which has not been disproved by aggregate data. For this reason, policies to raise average happiness must target much else besides economic growth. (2012: 86)

Inequality

The second point made by Layard et al. (2012) refers to inequality. Equality is important to politicians in a democracy since every vote is equally important come election time (at least in theory – voters in marginal constituencies or 'swing voters' may have greater marginal importance). The UK government's equality unit leads, according to the website, 'on issues relating to women, sexual orientation and transgender equality'. Equality is here being defined as freedom from discrimination. This definition of equality also includes equality for people with disabilities, minority ethnicities, religions or cultures. There is no doubt that discrimination leads to reduced well-being, and there would be few people who, in public at least, would argue for an increase in inequality although Kurt Vonnegut, in his short story, 'Harrison Bergeron', did imagine a dystopia in which dancers were hung with weights so that their motor performance was equal to people with average coordination, and very clever people were required to have a device in their heads to disrupt thinking to reduce their cognitive performance to the same level as people of average intelligence.

One way around this penalization of the more fortunate or well-endowed that Vonnegut was satirizing in his short story is to focus on equality for children, sometimes termed equality of opportunity, on the basis that children could all achieve their full potential if given equal opportunity.

Equality of income is a much more contentious issue than freedom from discrimination, partly because there are many who would argue that inequality here is inevitable and even good. One argument for maintaining social inequality is that the rich are rich as a reward for some profitable and therefore valuable social contribution – of course, this does not apply to those who are rich by inheritance although big fortunes often require several generations of wealth accumulation.

Another argument is the capitalist one, i.e. that we all benefit from capitalists because they invest their money in those socially valued projects that require large amounts of capital. For example, unless there had been very rich landlords in the 17th and 18th centuries in Europe, there would be fewer country houses for everyone, irrespective of their personal capital, to admire. Governments and non-profit-making institutions may amass capital, too, but are less willing to spend it on luxuries or frivolities even though some of the latter may turn out to be treasures for a future generation.

These economic arguments were contested by Marx and Engels in *Das Kapital* (Marx, 1961). They considered that capitalism inevitably resulted in a boom and bust economy. Capitalist endeavours require higher and higher levels of investment to maintain profits and that can only be achieved by reducing workers' wages or laying them off: or so it was argued, and is still argued back and forth. Engels (for it was he who wrote the later volumes of *Das Kapital*) developed a complex theory of surplus labour – that is the amount of labour available over and above the labour required to scratch a living – to explain this. A simpler way is that as profits fall, capitalists lay people off to try to push them back up, but this reduces the buying power of those in the market for their goods, fewer of which are sold, leading to a further fall in profits, and so on until, inevitably, a bust occurs. This can only be offset when productivity increases the income of the workers as well as the capitalists.

One of the arguments put forward by capitalists, or, as they are more often termed nowadays, free marketers, is the one that Adam Smith used: that a free market allows the greatest growth in Gross National Product, i.e. that when capitalists increase their own wealth, they also increase the wealth of those they employ. This crucially depends on the distribution of wealth in a society.

Marx argued 'to each according to their need', but the success of the 'dictatorship of the bourgeoisie' that Marx and Engels expected to be the last stage before this Communist utopia has proved to be unsuccessful unless rewards are made proportionate to output and not need. This inevitably leads to unequal distribution of income and thereby to social stratification. There is a strong link between social stratification and health, as shown in the moral force of communism or socialism which was given a voice by Marx in his descriptions of the plight of the working class, but the practical implementation of the dictatorship of the bourgeoisie that Marx thought would lead inevitably to a truly egalitarian state has been interpreted by many as an argument for inequality or, rather, as maintaining a link between income and industry. The ethical and political arguments between right and left wingers have prevented unbiased discussion of the link between social status and health and well-being. This is very clearly shown in Figure 5.1, taken from the second study of civil servants in the UK (Brunner et al., 1997).

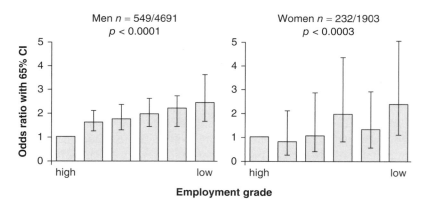

Figure 5.1 Adjusted odds ratios for metabolic syndrome by grade after adjustment for age and, in women, menopausal status

Note: P values are for trend tests across employment grade categories.

Source: Brunner, E. J., Marmot, M. G., Nanchahal, K., Shipley, M. J., Stansfield, S.A., Juneja, M., & Alberti, K. G. (1997). Social inequality in coronary risk: central obesity and the metabolic syndrome. Evidence from the Whitehall II study. *Diabetologia, 40*, 1341–1349.

Being in the lowest civil service grade was associated with a 2.5 times greater chance of developing metabolic syndrome (diabetes and heart disease), as the figure shows, with a proportionally falling risk as a person's civil service grade got higher. Marmot (2004) concluded that the underlying cause of this is job control, but it could also be education or simply income, leading to greater degrees of deprivation. The income of a clerical and support worker in the UK civil service is much higher in real terms than that of, say, a doctor in Africa. So it cannot be the absolute level of income that is the issue and, as we showed in a previous chapter, an increase in the national average or basic wage does not change these relationships. Hence, the issue is inequality of some kind or another. There have been numerous reports and an influential book (Wilkinson & Pickett, 2010) arguing that the fundamental inequality is income, but these publications have been hotly contested and, of course, the arguments against inequality all have the inevitable weakness that they are based on correlations. No one so far has taken a large and homogeneous group of people and given half of them an extra £50,000 a year for 10 years, comparing their health all the while with the less fortunate moiety. Even this experiment might be flawed by the emotional reactions of those who received this massive grant, since some people would probably resent the income and others would feel guilty about accepting it.

Even though a definitive experiment has not been carried out, the evidence for the well-being penalty created by inequality of income is so varied and so often replicated that it seems perverse not to accept it, even if the way in which inequality reduces well-being is still not established. As well as control, or autonomy, it has been suggested that resentment, anomie and pessimism might all be factors, and we will come back to these from the psychotherapist's viewpoint in Chapter 8. However, it is not obvious what a politician should do about it. Redistributing wealth against the grain of achievement, as Stalin did with the Kulaks, Mao Zedong did with the intellectuals and Mengistu Haile Maria and Robert Mugabe (who has since given Mengistu sanctuary) have done with land-owning farmers, has given rise to stories of atrocities, inefficient production, famine and suffering. Some revisionists question these conclusions and it is surprising to note that the average life expectancy of the Chinese jumped during the Cultural Revolution. Crushing one particular class or group of people might seem to be justifiable on utilitarian grounds if the majority benefit, but this is an emotionally repugnant argument. It may also be flawed. If crushing a few to help the many creates such a climate of fear even amongst the beneficiaries, it seems unlikely that well-being could possible increase.

Health inequalities

A less controversial approach to inequality has been to consider health inequality, without making any assumptions about how it is created. This is the approach taken by the UCL Health Inequalities Unit, chaired by Michael Marmot, which provided a 'strategic view of health inequalities post-2010', commissioned by the UK government (the report is called Fair Society, Healthy Lives). The approach was to look at mean age of death and other well-being indicators by area. There was surprising variation and when factors that co-varied with age at death were considered, income again emerged. People living in the poorest areas in England die, on average, seven years earlier and spend 17 more years of their lives living with a disability than people living in the richest neighbourhoods.

What should politicians do to increase well-being?

I think that individuals should be held responsible for their own emotional reactions. Of course, if their reactions become disordered, then people may need to seek help to regain control of their emotions – but they are responsible for seeking that help. Governments have a duty to ensure that it is provided, and I agree with Lord Layard that this means increasing the availability of therapy until it is sufficient to meet the needs of all those who seek it. I also think that governments should be held responsible for preventing corruption and combating oppression. Furthermore, society has a collective responsibility to care for vulnerable members and to control those members who might exploit, coerce or dupe their fellows.

Even if individuals, societies and governments all fulfil these duties, there are plenty of bouts of unhappiness or suffering that can still occur. How much can we hold politicians responsible for abating them?

Direct intervention to redistribute wealth is dictatorial. Indirect action through taxation to reduce wealth differentials is, it seems to me, a similar policy to adding duty on alcohol to reduce alcoholism. It may be effective but does not seem to be getting to the root cause.

Governments seem to me to be more successful when they focus on increasing freedoms rather than on increasing burdens. Increasing freedom does not mean laissez-faire economics: we are persuaded by those economists who think unplanned developed economies are subject to unnecessary boom and bust cycles if unregulated, and boom brings little increase in well-being whilst bust brings a considerable worsening of mental and physical health.

Franklin Roosevelt thought that there were four fundamental freedoms that politicians should address: freedom of speech and expression, freedom of worship, freedom from want and freedom from fear. These are all relevant to well-being, as we have seen in this chapter. These freedoms reflect a wider view of the responsibilities of government than increasing the GNP, but one of them, freedom from want, was the justification for focusing on GNP in the first place (other than the wartime reason of being able to produce war materials). Once want is not a major issue, the priorities shift, as I have indicated above. Hastings (2009), writing on behalf of the UN Economic and Social Commission for Asia and the Pacific Office of the United Nations, has argued that the shift should be towards peacefulness, fair circumstances for all people and long-term environmental sustainability.

6

The Extravert's Viewpoint

Suppose that you, dear reader, are a film director and that you have been asked to produce a short film about well-being in children. You want to start with an opening shot, creating the mood. Obviously, you would want to have children in it. You would probably show them laughing or at least smiling, since happiness and well-being are so closely linked. They would need to look healthy, and probably be running or involved in some active game, to show that they are healthy, since health and well-being are also closely linked. Their environment would probably be a natural one, free of grime and overcrowded buildings, given the links between access to parks and well-being (Douglas, 2012). Their clothes would look new and not be torn or mended to indicate that these children came from families that did not know material want. Something though would still be missing from the shot if that was all there was. To really convey well-being, of the kind that we dream our children and grandchildren will have, you, as the director, would want to show the children being happy in interaction – playing a game together, for example. You would want to imply that these were children with their friends, having a good time.

If you wanted to highlight the happy children, you might also show another child, alone, somewhere to the margin of the picture. Perhaps she would have her head hanging, looking pensive. Perhaps she would be reading.

The words 'extravert' and 'introvert' were invented by Jung but have passed into our language. Most of us would be inclined to think of the happy, running children as extraverts, and the shy, solitary child as an introvert. Extraverts are more sociable, and according to recent happiness researchers, extraversion is linked to happiness. In a long-term follow-up study (Gale et al., 2013), extraversion at age 16 and age 28 was significantly associated with well-being at over 60 years of age, although the association was weak (see Figure 6.1). Neuroticism was also linked, but the authors concluded that this was mediated by anxiety. 'Neuroticism' is a measure of proneness to anxiety. Other studies have come to similar conclusions (Kokko et al., 2013; Wilt et al., 2012).

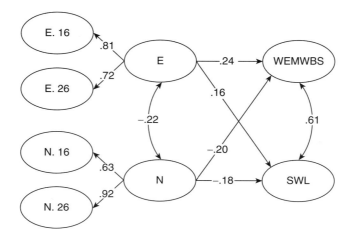

Figure 6.1 Structural diagram for the main effects between personality and well-being

Notes: E.16 = extraversion measured at age 16; E.26 = extraversion measured at age 26;
N.16 = neuroticism measured at age 16; N.26 = neuroticism measured at age 26. E = extraversion;
N = neuroticism; WEMWBS = Warwick–Edinburgh Mental Wellbeing Scale total score; SWL =
Satisfaction with Life total score. Parameter estimates are standardized and significant at a
minimum p < .05.

Source: Gale et al., 2013, Neuroticism and extraversion in youth predict mental wellbeing and life
satisfaction 40 years later. *Journal of Research in Personality, 47(6)*, 687–697.

Extraversion

Carl Jung (1923) coined the term extravert when he began to establish his international reputation as a psychotherapist. As a much younger man, he had conducted
experiments using a machine, called a psycho-galvanometer, that would later become
the core of the 'lie detector' and a staple in laboratory studies of anxiety. He was
using the free association technique developed by the English philosopher Francis
Galton, that was also being used to great effect in the neighbouring country of Austria
(Jung was Swiss) by Sigmund Freud. Participants had to say a word that was associated for them with a word given by the experimenter. Their sweatiness was measured
by the psycho-galvanometer at the same time. When the stimulus word triggered a
word association that was emotional, the response was often delayed and the subject
sweated more. Jung described what was being evoked as a 'complex'. Complex formation was not purely sexual – a point of difference with Freud – and not even linked to
the remote past – another difference with Freud. One participant sweated a lot when
given the word 'floor'. When Binswanger, who was conducting this particular experiment, asked the participant what it meant, the man said that his stove had recently

caught fire and not only destroyed itself but also the floor on which it stood, requiring an expensive rebuilding job as well as making him feel that he had only just escaped a much more serious fire (Peterson & Jung, 1907). Perhaps it was this experiment that set Binswanger on the path of existential therapy, which considers the importance of current life difficulties rather than past traumata.

Jung and his co-workers thought that there might be another reason for a delayed response than that of emotional conflict, which they described as follows: 'Individuals with good powers of introspection often affirm that they could not respond quickly, because of the sudden crowding into consciousness of a number of words among which they could find none suitable for the reaction' (Jung, 1923: 190).

Jung later built a typology of 'attitudes' on the basis of introspection, coining the term 'introvert' for people who distrusted the outside world and preferred to spend time thinking or focusing on their own bodily sensations. Introverts were contrasted with 'extraverts' who felt comfortable with their environment, were outgoing and preferred not to dwell too much or too morbidly on themselves (Jung, 1923). Jung thought that he was breaking entirely new ground by focusing on feelings or affects, although commentators since have seen links with the Galenic temperament that Jung specifically disavowed, and also links with Nietzsche's distinction between introspective Apollonians and outgoing Dionysians.

The distinction between introversion and extraversion has proved a durable one. It is one of the big five temperamental characteristics that many psychologists consider to be fundamental to what they term 'personality'. Quite contrary to Jung's idea that it was not related to temperament, extraversion has a strong hereditary contribution, at least as extraversion is nowadays typified on standard 'scales' or questionnaires. Jung had already signalled that he thought extraversion was somehow healthier than introversion, and this attitude has grown to such an extent that a recent book, *Quiet*, has become popular because its author has defended the social value of introverts (Cain, 2012).

Social advantages of extraversion

Extraverts have higher well-being and job satisfaction, especially in China (Zhai et al., 2012), where work is even more team-based than in other parts of the world. One reason may be that extraverts are confident about reaching out to other people for support. When someone is feeling down, talking to other people may help, whether or not that someone is an extravert or an introvert. But this may only be true for introverts if they know that there is a friendly person present, whereas extraverts can feel better after discussion even if there is no one present that they know to be supportive (Augustine & Hemenover, 2008). As a result, extraverts are more likely to have social support than introverts (Chay, 1993).

Extraverts have more social connections than introverts, and some studies suggest that the number of social connections is what matters for well-being and that it is social connectedness that links extraversion to well-being (Lee et al., 2008).

Looking some more at social connectedness

I introduced this chapter with an image of children laughing and playing together. It was an image of happiness, but it might also have been an image of the human animal or what it is like to be human; this is one way of illustrating what Heidegger called 'Dasein' – existence. Heidegger unpicked this everyday German word, pointing out that it was derived from 'da' and 'sein' – being there. The 'there' for all of us, he pointed out, is being with others, 'Mitsein'. When we think of people, we are actually thinking of people inextricably connected to other people and not a bunch of individual units. Each of us is connected to a family, a culture, a body and an environment, created or modified by people. Being connected, including being socially connected, is therefore our default state. In fact, I have argued that it goes further than this, and that our brains are connected by a constant traffic of non-verbal communication, just as our computers are interconnected wirelessly by an internet connection. Even when we are alone, we are, or so I have argued, running over our stories about other people and the stories that they have told about our social world and about us (Tantam, 2009).

Connections with other people may be irretrievably broken through marginalization or exclusion or simply 'otherness'. People with stigmatizing health problems, people who are shunned or members of undervalued minorities are at risk of experiencing this. Native Australians living in predominantly new Australian areas have three times the level of depression and anxiety as new Australians, for example (Cunningham & Paradies, 2012).

Relationships

Being connected to others may be our default state, but the connections transfer emotions that are not always pleasant. Connections solidify into ties, or positions, in which one person may be dominant and another subordinate. Imperceptible connections solidify into social relationships. Social relationships are tied into many, if not most, of our activities, and not all of these are pleasant. Relationships are normally complex, often with positive and negative feelings, joys and resentments, woven into them. They wax and wane, becoming more or less intimate. They are linked to work or to family life. They have many purposes, including performing tasks collaboratively, having sex, bringing up children, playing games, artistic expression through dance or music, conducting ceremonies, and fighting or warfare. Relationships are maintained in our mind's eye, even when the person or persons with whom we have the relationship are absent. Some people seem less good at maintaining these virtual relationships (variously called mental representations, inner objects, other-person narratives) and are more likely to get lonely on their own as a result. Loneliness is what people experience when they are missing out on the emotional benefits of social relationship. Loneliness may occur as people get older, often because of a combination of bereavement and a lack of relationship development and maintenance. However, people may also be actively pushed out of social groups, a process often termed marginalization or social exclusion, and feel lonely as a result. A lack of social relationships may be put down to a lack of opportunity or the intrinsic unlikeability of the lonely person, in which case the emotional consequences are likely to be more negative.

Psychological and social research can rarely capture this kind of complexity, relying on very crude categorizations of the effects of relationships on happiness and health in terms of social support, often restricting this even further to the relief of negative emotions through social relationships and social integration and relief of the negative consequences of social relationships (Cohen, 2004). We often think of relationships as being most important to our well-being, but intimate relationships, which many of us would consider particularly linked to well-being, have both positive and negatives. Negative consequences of close relationships are well known to psychotherapists, but the positive consequences (which most health psychologists focus on) often involve large scale studies or the totality of each person's extended relationships, their social networks, in which the negative relationships for a minority of people in a few bad but crucial relationships get lost.

A further, final contribution of social connections is through the increase in personal efficacy that they permit (Obrien et al., 2012). We shall call the latter 'social integration'.

Social support

In previous chapters, we have noted that most people have some negative feelings during the course of a day, even if overall they rate their day or themselves as happy. One factor that makes positive feelings outweigh negative ones is that the latter are reduced in duration or severity by social interaction with positively inclined others (Chay, 1993).

Social support enhances well-being primarily by reducing the effects of negative experiences on happiness and health. Socially isolated people, like other socially isolated mammals, have a greater vulnerability to depression, blunted immune response and higher levels of adrenal 'stress hormones' (Cacioppo et al., 2011). So, at a very basic level, kindly contact with others may reduce negative feelings and enhance social interaction. This contact may be physical as in stroking or grooming (Voos et al., 2012) or verbal, as in soothing or merely uncritical and attentive listening. Relationship quality is more important than the number of different relationships in mediating this effect (Leach et al., 2012).

Social integration

Social integration means belonging to a social group, especially in the sense of having a role, place or value. Its absence leads to what Weiss (1973) termed social loneliness, as opposed to the emotional loneliness that is associated with a lack of intimacy. Social integration enhances positive feelings, possibly mediated via the dopaminergic receptors that are associated with reward.

Negative effects of social interaction

Having social support and being socially integrated each contribute independently to well-being and health, through decreasing negative feelings and increasing positive feelings and as a source of practical help, but social interaction is not always positive.

One of the biggest sources of negative experience is other people, and negative experience peaks in middle age, possibly accounting for the finding that well-being is greatest in the youngest and oldest members of the population (Darbonne et al., 2012). Interpersonal conflict makes a substantial contribution to increasing negative feelings (Whisman & Baucom, 2012) and therefore reducing well-being and health, just as social support decreases them. As we have seen, older people make more efforts to reduce conflict, and younger people rely more than the middle-aged on sexual relationships as a means of reducing conflict and therefore depression (Whitton & Kuryluk, 2012). Social support therefore has most impact for the middle-aged, although supportive relationships in infancy seem to increase the ability of adults to make use of what social support is available.

Conflict, threat, humiliation, marginalization, control and demand are among the negative aspects of social interactions that give rise to negative feelings. Submission, frustration and withholding reduce positive feelings. When either set of social interactions becomes the most common in a relationship, happiness and health both deteriorate.

Depression is recognized throughout the world as the illness that most reduces quality of life and well-being. It has a strong hereditary component, but identical twins, who share the same genes, may sometimes be discordant for depression. Kendler (Kendler & Halberstadt, 2012) interviewed women who were identical twins and in whom one twin had become depressed and one not. Although life events sometimes explained why one twin and not the other had become depressed, this was rare. The most frequent explanation was that the depressed twin had the misfortune to have a bad relationship with a partner.

Formative early experience

Identical twins often share the same early environment as well as the same genes. Kendler's analysis, cited in the previous paragraph, does not distinguish between the two. 'Blank slate' theories minimize inborn differences, arguing that every newborn is a blank slate onto which experience writes. The future happiness and health of the identical twins in the Kendler study would, according to blank slate theorists, have been due to their shared early experience. Kendler and his co-workers have provided evidence against this in another study. In that, they find evidence for a single combination of genes that is conserved when passed down from one generation to the next, and which accounts for a substantial amount of the differences between one person's well-being and that of another (Keyes et al., 2010).

One possible candidate for this general factor of well-being is oxytocin. Oxytocin is one of the hormones involved in the feeling that one loves another person so much that one could eat them up. It is at its highest in a mother when she holds her baby, with whom she has bonded. It peaks too during the early phase of a romantic attachment (Schneiderman et al., 2012). Oxytocin reduces negative feelings (Smith & Wang, 2012), increases empathy and social intelligence (Yamasue et al., 2012), increases the responsiveness of infants to their fathers, if those fathers have been given oxytocin (Weisman et al., 2012) and increases sensitivity to a mother's disgust in adult daughters who remain close to their mothers (Huffmeijer et al., 2012) where the daughters have been given oxytocin snuff.

The gene for the enzyme that produces oxytocin, and the gene for the receptor that is triggered by it, exists in different forms in the population (Walum et al., 2012), which means that a human population is likely to have some people who are less responsive to oxytocin. Evolutionary psychology suggests that, as these people are not dying out, there must be some evolutionary benefit that offsets their greater difficulties in forming social relationships. We will come back to this apparent anomaly later when we discuss extraversion.

Studies of rats suggest that the extent to which mothers lick or groom their offspring also modulates the oxytocin responsiveness of their offspring's brains (Champagne et al., 2001); in other words, maternal contact and comfort acts alongside genetics to influence later oxytocin responsiveness. The human equivalents of licking and grooming in rats are hugging, kissing, stroking and soothing vocalizations. These are used to express affection but also to calm. Their effects on well-being are therefore to increase positive feelings and diminish negative ones.

The diminution of negative feelings, particularly of anxiety, has been the focus of many psychoanalytically derived theories of the importance of early experience. Attachment theory is one of the most systematic of these. The relationship of oxytocin to psychological attachment is unclear. Rather than oxytocin, the transmitter most often implicated in the impact of early experience on anxiety is serotonin (Kiser et al., 2012). Early experience of how one's mother copes with one's anxiety – often experimentally induced by a period of separation from the mother – does correlate with many aspects of well-being during infancy and early childhood, though the links with how anxiety is handled in adulthood have often been asserted but not satisfactorily proved. Maternal depression (Turney, 2012) and a lack of social confidence, or shyness, are both linked to diminished relationship quality and well-being in later life (Rowsell & Coplan, 2012). These links may not be emotional in nature but relate to social competence. Infant care-givers who are not depressed tell their infants stories about feelings and social relationships, and, in middle childhood, peers also contribute to each other's social competence by re-telling stories about what has gone on in the playground. This social competence has an important impact on adulthood as understanding significant other persons is an important element in close relationships (Finkenauer & Righetti, 2011). Cognitive disadvantages, for example in working memory, may also accumulate, affecting educational attainment and therefore well-being in adulthood. Poverty and disadvantage may also accrue and diminish well-being and health in later life (Shonkoff & Garner, 2012).

7

The Spiritual Viewpoint

In the last chapter, I considered the limitations of well-being as an explanation of what makes life worthwhile. Some of this shortfall is taken up by the additional scope of the term 'living well'. Living well for most people requires other people and not just oneself to be taken into account. Connectedness to others emerged in the last chapter as an important mediating factor between extraversion, what I called well-being capital, and well-being itself. Durkheim (2008) argued that social connectedness is fundamental to religion, too, and Augustine of Hippo (Augustine, 2009) attributed the derivation of the word 'religio' to the Latin word, ligare, to bind, implying that religion binds people together (the etymology is, however, disputed).

Religion is grounded in spirituality, but there are many spiritual people who would not define themselves as religious. Even so, they might claim that the root of their spirituality is their connectedness to something greater than themselves – for example, nature, mankind, the universe, philosophy even or science or poetry. Perhaps this is not quite enough for a spiritual experience. There also has to be an element of self-effacement and an element of dedication to the greater good. People sometimes say that 'just living for me is not enough to give my life meaning'. This missing dimension is often called 'spirituality' and I will look at the relationship between spirituality and living well in more detail in this chapter.

What Einstein thought

Living well does not always mean following Bentham's (1876) dictum and making as many people as possible happy. Many people consider that they have lived well, even though they have been dedicated to fighting, subjugating or even killing adversaries. There have been periods in history when the number of people one was responsible for killing was linked to other people's esteem. However, there are many others who would consider that a life spent killing people is not a life well spent, even if the killings are not criminal but state-sanctioned.

Here, for example, is what Einstein (1930) thought about the military:

> This topic brings me to that worst outcrop of herd life, the military system, which I abhor ... This plague-spot of civilization ought to be abolished with all possible speed. Heroism on command, senseless violence, and all the loathsome nonsense that goes by the name of patriotism – how passionately I hate them! (ibid., p. 2)

Despite this, Einstein recommended to Franklin Roosevelt that the USA develop an atomic bomb before Germany did. It is ironic that, despite his passionate rejection of military life, he was therefore indirectly implicated – even though he refused to join the Manhattan project – in the deaths at Hiroshima and Nagasaki.

Einstein's position involves some degree of self-deception, just like the rest of us when we buy cheap eggs, not thinking about battery chickens; cheap clothes, not thinking about child labour; cheap foreign holidays, not thinking of environmental damage; or, as in Einstein's case, benefit from the freedoms that soldiers have fought for on our behalf. It presupposes some degree of moral luck: had he not become as famous as he did, and so had not been visiting Princeton at the start of the war, he might have still been in Berlin and thereby caught up in the horrors of the Holocaust. Would his view about the military that fought the Fascists have remained the same then? If we are not faced with difficult decisions, we can assume that we would have made the right ones without having to put this to the test.

In the paragraph that follows the one on militarism, Einstein (1930) sets out his faith in spirituality:

> The most beautiful experience we can have is the mysterious. It is the fundamental emotion that stands at the cradle of true art and true science. Whoever does not know it and can no longer wonder, no longer marvel, is as good as dead, and his eyes are dimmed. It was the experience of mystery – even if mixed with fear – that engendered religion. (ibid., p. 3)

Many of us find this a much easier sentiment to believe in. No one can be harmed by a belief in beauty or mystery, we think (although religions have provoked a great many wars).

Einstein, in his brief article, seems to pin living well to his work, his creativity and the beauty of the mysterious. Surveys regularly show that people with a strong religious faith (a kind of spirituality, as Einstein indicates) are happier and healthier than the general population.

Spirituality and connectedness to other people

Why should spirituality involve connectedness to other people? One could imagine someone – a mountaineer, say, or a lone yachtswoman or a hermit – who has honed their personal survival skills to the point that they do not need other people, but get their transcendental experience from reaching the summits of the highest mountains, or crossing the widest oceans, or being with god. But even they will have a support team, a family who has at the very least given them the wherewithal to be so self-sufficient, and lovers, friends, children, employers, staff members or fans, all of whose well-being is linked to theirs.

A very self-centred person might still say that all of these other people are being repaid for their efforts either in money or in reflected glory, but such an answer reflects the inevitability of considering other people's well-being when seeking one's own. Of course, it is possible that other people do not exist, or at least so philosophers have supposed. However, Wittgenstein's answer is the one that most people naturally give to the solipsism problem: 'My attitude towards him is an attitude towards a soul. I am not of the opinion that he has a soul' (Wittgenstein, 1958: II, iv).

In other words, we do not need to justify the existence of other people any more than we do our own. We develop our consciousness of ourselves, taking for granted that we and other people are part of an existing world that we are discovering.

Robert Nozick (1974) imagined an 'experience machine' that we have already considered in Chapter 1. It would provide delicious, if deceptive, experience to those within it. He thought that most people, woken up after a period in the machine, and told that their life was virtual, would want to go back to 'real' living. He intuitively thought that most people would think that life that was not real was somehow lessened, even though in the machine what they experience is indistinguishable from real life in every respect but that they felt constantly happy and healthy.

What would be missing for those in the 'experience machine' would be a sense of the impact of their own actions on other people (Appiah, 2008), such as their capacity to cause real harm. Nozick's (1974) experience machine has been all but realized: continuous computer gaming and drug misuse do seem to spread unreality over real life, especially in young people whose hold on reality may not be particularly secure. Re-enactments of game scenarios in real life can then lead to real people being shot, killed or wounded with the perpetrator remaining emotionally detached.

Why does it matter that our actions have a real effect? Surely, life would be simpler if, whatever we do, no one would deserve to be punished and no one would get angry or resentful about our actions? The experience machine could, presumably, be programmed to ensure this. But, even so, it seems likely that a machine user would conclude that their apparent actions in the machine have been 'meaningless' as soon as they realize that real people, real events and real happenings are not influenced by them (perhaps with the exception that they might seem meaningful as 'practice', but that would presuppose that they were practice for the 'real thing').

I agree with Spinoza (Spinoza & Wolf, 1910) that this preference for the real rather than the made up or artificial, however seductive that is, is what constitutes the basis for spirituality (this is not to say that we do not believe that people may be mistaken or even deluded about what is real, and that their spiritual impulse can never be based on a flawed foundation).

How can we know the real?

Knowing that we are having a real experience, rather than being in the experience machine, comes through our ability to act on others, and therefore through our connection with others. A very good experience machine could simulate this. So our connection has to involve us knowing that others are subjects in themselves, and not a mere simulation, just as we are a subject in ourselves: as Buber said, to have an I–Thou relationship with another person and not an I–it one. Experiencing this already takes us out of our ordinary world, the day world as Heidegger calls it, and into a heightened sense of awareness of other people. But how can we be sure that we are not misleading ourselves?

Many philosophical attempts to tackle the solipsism problem have not solved it to everyone's satisfaction. One possible reason is that the evidence for other people being there, and us being connected to them, is not evidence at all in that it is not based on facts that we can check or reason about. It is a consequence of how we are constructed.

I have proposed (Tantam, 2009) that our brains are directly influenced by other brains through the to-and-fro traffic of nonverbal communication that passes between one person and another, but outside their conscious awareness. Examples of this are that we turn our gaze on what other people are looking at without realizing it, and our facial expressions mirror those of other people around us, leading to a kind of emotional contagion or empathy.

If this 'interbrain' hypothesis is correct – and obviously I think that it is – then our brains act and react to other brains well before each brain can provide the substrate for a mind to call into doubt whether or not the other brain is there. The idea that we automatically take account of other people is not new. David Hume and his friend Adam Smith (2002) both supposed that sympathy (nowadays we reserve this term for 'compassion' and would use empathy for what Hume and Smith called sympathy) exists spontaneously between people, leading us to take them into account.

The interbrain, or empathy, or sympathy, whatever we want to call it, provides an emotional connection between people that is the touchstone of what we are calling 'the real'. Often, people associate moments of heightened empathy with another person, usually at times of high emotion, as feeling a heightened sense of reality.

Spirituality

Feeling really connected to another person (or another animal), often at a time of heightened emotion, may be a necessary condition of spiritual experience, but it is not enough. Wittgenstein thought that another element was the failure of language to describe it, and this would fit with our idea that it is an experience that happens before we have time to put it into words. Another necessary condition may be that we go beyond what we thought we knew about ourselves and our world (the previous sentence is a good example of the failure of language – for how can we possibly go beyond ourselves and still be ourselves?). Curiously, two words that are normally taken to be antonyms equally apply to this going beyond. We may become aware of unexpected depths in ourselves, of the immanent in ourselves, and that may turn out to be what makes us experience ourselves as subjects rather than, say, machines or people living in machines. Husserl (1967) imagined this process as involving removing our preconceptions about

ourselves and replacing them with less biased perception, a process he called reduction, and thought that we might reveal a kind of pure or unsullied ego that he called the
transcendental ego. He called it transcendental even though it begins as immanence,
according to the French philosopher, Michel Henry (2008). It is transcendental because
discovering our own transcendental ego brings with it a connection with the transcendental ego in other human beings.

The going beyond our own boundaries process can go exactly the other way round
too. In throwing ourselves outwards into nature, or into a relationship with a god, or
even into a relationship with family or some other social institution, we can discover
what 'really matters to us', as people say. We can discover, in other words, what is
immanent in ourselves, once we are driven to set aside small decisions and short-lived
emotions.

Organized religion

Organized religion is one important outlet of spirituality. It provides an additional
dimension of socialization and participation in community, and so provides many of
the relationship benefits considered in the last chapter. There are many who argue that
this or that faith guarantees that life will be lived well, and some that promise eternal
well-being. This last claim is difficult to trump, but, so far as I am concerned, such claims
are counter-intuitive, but fit so well with wishful thinking and credulousness as to make
them doubtful. I find myself gob-smacked by the paradoxes in showing that identity can
be continuous from one life to the next or from one life to an afterlife. Without such continuity, claims for immortality are obviously considerably weakened and indeed trivial.
There is no doubt that the elements of the human body persist and are reincorporated
into other substances, including other bodies. Nor is there any doubt that memories, and
memorials, keep a person alive in a certain way. Arguably, a person might consider that
following a formula to obtain immortality is the best way of living, even if the formula
requires them to be very unhappy and unhealthy. Like Pascal, I question whether anyone
can know after such questions. Pascal (1995) argued from this that if we cannot know, we
can gamble, and that we should gamble on immortality. I disagree with this, since even
if gambling on immortality is a sensible reading of the odds, it takes no account of the
risks of losing one's stake. Pascal did not think that there was a stake, but there clearly is:
it's the possibility of self-deception.

I will not be considering the benefits of one faith over another since I am not convinced that any offer committed and thoughtful adherents any advantage over the adherents of other faiths – although I note that there are many faiths that have lived and died
within historical times that were clearly opposed to well-being. For example, the Skopsoi,
a sect of old Russian believers, demanded of their most committed members that they
have their external genitalia completely removed (although it appears that very few took
up this invitation). The Skopsoi survived as a group for centuries, providing a disproportionate number of members of the financial industry in Tsarist Russia, but I think it
doubtful they could make a case for offering their adherents the greatest well-being, and

it is difficult, in retrospect, to think that they lived better by cutting of their genitalia. Being expected to castrate oneself, with its inevitable health consequences, must make the Skopsoi an unusually unrewarding group to commit to.

Advice for living

Organized religions have created bodies of spiritual guidance – some oral and some written – and I will occasionally refer to these as a source of wisdom that everyone may usefully draw on, irrespective of their faith. However, I recognize the dangers of misunderstanding when doing this. Most wisdom requires some hermeneutic work before it can be applied to one's own times or one's own world, and this work is less likely to be effective when working in another tradition.

Ritual observance

Spirituality may simply be a dimension of experience, but is often also created and refreshed in ritual observance. Such observances have several functions. One of them is to ward off evil. The tenebrae services of the Christian church, or the dancing step of the child who avoids standing on the cracks in the pavement, are examples. Rituals may create connections between participants. Perhaps most importantly, they may be meditational, providing a route by which participants can be in contact with a deity or an enhanced awareness of reality, by means of dance, music, prayer, offerings and religious images.

Behavioural manifestations of spirituality provide a means of maintaining a connection even after a real connection has died. Victor Frankl, the originator of logotherapy and famous for finding meaning even in the bleak surroundings of a Nazi concentration camp, said Kaddish every morning from the moment of his incarceration until he died. I do not know whether he said Kaddish for his first wife or for his parents or his sister, all of whom died in the camps. But he did say this:

> In a position of utter desolation, when man cannot express himself in positive action, when his only achievement may consist in enduring his sufferings in the right way – an honourable way – in such a position man can, through loving contemplation of the image he carries of his beloved, achieve fulfilment. For the first time in my life I was able to understand the meaning of the words, 'The angels are lost in perpetual contemplation of an infinite glory'. (Frankl, 1984: 31)

Being a member of a religious communion or community has, as the words communion and community themselves suggest, similarities with being in a family or a close relationship. These effects seem to spread beyond those directly involved in the communion. Church- (and presumably temple-, mosque- or synagogue-) going creates one kind of social capital, and people who live in communities where church-going is frequent have higher well-being than people who live in areas of low church-going, even if they do not go to church themselves. Research into the relationship between religion and well-being suggests that belonging to a religious community is associated with better health rather than if not (Kark et al., 1996). As Michael Argyle has pointed out, this does not clear up one of the fundamental questions of causation: does religion cause happiness or vice versa? Kleinman has suggested that the main benefit of organized religion is that it provides social contact and strong social networks. The benefits of church attendance in terms of increasing subjective well-being were, in one study, strongest in those who were single, old, retired or in poor health (Moberg & Taves, 1965). One explanation is that churches provide social contact for those who would otherwise be marginalized, and Argyle suggested that religious practice engenders well-being by: providing a supportive atmosphere including intimacy and self-disclosure, allowing followers to feel close to God (which allows God to be used as a coping mechanism), providing followers with firm beliefs or 'existential certainty', and promoting good health amongst followers by discouraging drinking, smoking and promiscuous sex. These traditional certainties may now be breaking down (Lewis & Cruise, 2006).

Studies of the adherents of organized religions all over the world seem to report similar levels of well-being. Presumably, if there was one religion which was far superior in terms of the happiness it bestowed on its followers, then this religion would spread and become dominant. In the same way, presumably any religions which do not engender feelings of well-being are unlikely to catch on and will not have many followers (although one wonders about the Skopsoi). To use a Darwinian analogy, there is a 'survival of the fittest' in terms of religions and a 'natural selection' occurring to weed out any unsuccessful varieties. And ironically, with similarity to comparisons of different therapies, the relative similarity of different religions in terms of the well-being they produce probably relates to the quality of social contact with other humans which these faiths encourage, rather than to the particular nature of the divinity being worshipped.

Secular values

It has been a natural progression for Seligman and other positive psychologists to move from considering what makes people feel happy to the determinants of well-being, and then on to spirituality – just as I have followed the trajectory in this book. Peterson and Seligman in a substantial work (Peterson & Seligman, 2004) concluded that there were six core values: wisdom and knowledge; courage; love and humanity; justice; temperance; and spirituality and transcendence. They also concluded that there were 24 identifiable personal strengths that could be cultivated to live out these values as well as possible.

This 'virtues in action' approach was based on polls of professionals and on a literature review, and it has not stood up well to empirical testing (Shryack et al., 2010), although it has been tested in different countries (Alex Linley et al., 2007) and age groups (Weber et al., 2013). One reason might be that people have very different values, even if cultural institutions, like churches or schools, tend to teach the same ones. Prescriptive or official values that people pay lip service to may be very different to the values that each individual holds to in their personal life.

Spirituality and psychotherapy

It seems from conversations with professionals that many counsellors and psychotherapists do see their work as connected with spirituality in some way: that although counselling or psychotherapy may not be a spiritual activity in itself, by relieving emotional suffering, counsellors and psychotherapists may enable their clients to be more aware of the spiritual in their lives. Those holding this view would consider that one benefit of counselling or psychotherapy is that it allows a person's spirituality to flourish. Note that this is not the same as saying that a person has a beneficial spiritual life, if such a term even applies, but that a person might have a more spiritual life, for good or ill. The distinction is analogous to that between happiness and the pursuit of happiness. Having the opportunity and the hope of pursuing happiness does not guarantee happiness, but it is a prerequisite of it. Similarly, having enough peace of mind to become aware of the spiritual elements in life does not guarantee an active spiritual life, but it is a prerequisite of it. It does not appear as though anyone has yet considered spirituality as a beneficial outcome of counselling or psychotherapy in any study. It is an area fraught with pitfalls. We would, for example, expect that scientology would be one of the more successful interventions if a concern about spiritual development was taken to be a good outcome, but it was precisely because the UK government of the day wanted to discourage scientology without discouraging psychotherapy that the UK psychotherapy registration process was begun.

Spirituality and healing

Spiritual healing is the predecessor of psychotherapy. In cultures where spirituality is strong, spiritual healing methods are often preferred to Western psychotherapy. Outcome studies show that spiritual healing can be as effective as Westernized therapy in relieving depression and anxiety. Some of the therapeutic factors may be the same. Spiritual healing may be more acceptable to some people than Western forms of therapy, and it seems particularly appropriate for the passages in life or from life to death that are associated with religious ceremonials. Like other effective healing practices, spiritual healing can also be upsetting and even harmful. Many spiritual healing practices attribute illness to the presence in the body, or the influence over the body, of harmful spirits. These may gain entry because a person does something that makes them vulnerable, such as travelling by sea or sleeping under a tree (these and subsequent examples are taken from my own study of exorcism in Zanzibar), through a failure to observe a religious practice or ceremony, through the malice of the recently dead or though the malice of witches or wizards (who often turn out to be neighbours with whom the affected person is in dispute). All of these situations would also be recognized as stressful ones in the West: even sorcery becomes understandable if we identify it as bullying at work by a bad boss or hassle at home over a joint boundary with a stroppy neighbour. Methods of spiritual healing may involve purgation (to release the spirits), being touched by something holy (holy water, a relic, a religious symbol of some kind) or drinking something holy. In Islamic healing, this is often a decoction of an apposite scripture written in turmeric and then washed off into a bottle. More persistent spirits may require more emotionally demanding methods such as exorcism or substitution. In the latter, the spirit or principle of illness is transferred into an inanimate object and then manipulated in some way to make it harmless.

Does leading a spiritual life lead to well-being?

So what is the evidence that having a spiritual dimension in life is necessary for well-being? And could we have this without feeling connected to others, or is living well, which we are defining as living so that other people's well-being is enhanced as well as our own, the route to the greatest well-being? Many wise people have come to this conclusion. We have already quoted Bentham and the economist Richard Layard. Mark Twain (1935) had a related idea. He wrote: 'The best way to cheer yourself is to try to cheer someone else up.' (ibid., p. 310). Charlotte Brontë also thought that connectedness was essential to happiness, although not for altruistic reasons. Gaskell (1909) quotes her as saying towards the end of her life: 'Happiness quite unshared can scarcely be called happiness; it has no taste.' (ibid., p. 125) Bronte's comment may be particularly apposite to conscious feelings of happiness, since she was probably using taste to refer to a perception or conscious reflection on sensation.

There have been no direct studies of affective empathy and well-being, although one study has shown that imagining losing someone close leads people to be more alert to nonverbal communication and motivated to increase their social connectedness (Gray et al., 2011). However, connectedness is one of the factors that distinguishes nonagenarians from younger people in many studies, suggesting a link between connectedness and health. Connectedness was the last stage of life that Eric Erikson's widow added to the posthumous edition of *Childhood and Society*, which was subsequently re-titled *The Life Cycle Completed* (Erikson & Erikson, 1997).

Positive psychology, one study suggests, partly works through its effects on connectedness. Happy people who do not show happiness on their faces are likely to become less happy with time, along with feeling more disconnected from other people, than equally happy people who smile at others (Mauss et al., 2011). It would be unusual to be a positive person and not smile at others, of course, because there is also a link between extraversion and a positive hedonic balance, as we noted in Chapter 3. In fact, even introverts can become happier by behaving like extraverts (Zelenski et al., 2012).

In one study (Lo et al., 2011), spirituality and connectedness were associated with greater well-being and less physical suffering during terminal care, and in a meta-analysis a correlation between reduced mortality in healthy people (but not people with an illness) and greater spiritual or religious involvement was also found (Chida et al., 2009), but the authors of the meta-analysis question whether there was a bias against publishing studies in which there was no, or a negative, correlation. Positive feelings are associated with spiritual experiences, hope and a sense of life having meaning (Wnuk & Marcinkowski, 2012), but which way these associations go is not clear.

Connectedness does not always lead to a feeling of enhancement. If we are not satisfied with our lives, then that dissatisfaction can be increased through the same social comparison process that makes any social inequality galling. Social network users are vulnerable to this kind of adverse social comparison, especially if their networks include 'non-friends' (Chou & Edge, 2012). People with face-to-face friends may experience this less, although there is some research evidence that women's friendships may involve an evaluative element that can lead to an increase in negative feelings following contact with friends. Too many Facebook friends may reduce rather than increase self-esteem.

Even if we assume that connectedness is a requirement for well-being, this does not necessarily mean that we have to treat well those to whom we are connected. We could imagine a tyrant who is closely connected to others but treats them badly. Mao Zedung, for example, is believed to have instigated purges, torture and starvation that killed millions of people. He is also reported to have had many children whom he abandoned. According to two commentators (Courtois & Kramer, 1999): 'Mao Zedong was so powerful that he was often known as the Red Emperor ... the violence he erected into a whole system far exceeds any national tradition of violence that we might find in China.'

Mao lived to the age of 82, but his health had deteriorated before that. He had two heart attacks, developed a neurodegenerative disorder and suffered with several sexually transmitted diseases. He reportedly had periods of worry and unhappiness, when he would take to his bed, sometimes for weeks. He suffered from insomnia and took sleeping pills. Hence, it does not seem that he had as much well-being as many other octagenarians. Stalin and Hitler, too, had sleep problems and minor but troubling ailments.

Perhaps ensuring the well-being of others, and living well, is linked to personal well-being, especially as one gets older, when spiritual well-being becomes more important. It is likely that Mao was born with a normal interbrain connection – with a normal degree of empathy for other people, in other words – but that he learned to control his empathy according to whether or not it suited his political goals. Towards the end of his life, his personal physician reported that Mao slept with as many young women as possible in the belief that this would keep him young, but despite being told by his physician that he had STDs and would be passing them on to these apparently willing victims, he refused treatment. Ordinary people can suspend their empathy too: soldiers can persuade themselves, for example, that rape in warfare is normal, even natural (Baaz & Stern, 2009), whilst blanking off the terror that they cause the victim, whether male or female, when they rape them.

Mao, Stalin and Hitler were clearly out of the ordinary in being able to insulate themselves against the suffering of so many people. Perhaps the only way to do this, or the only way to stop being a soldier and to become a normal, moral citizen again, is to live 'being a soldier' in a kind of unreal world in which the violence takes place, dissociated from 'real life'. This would be like being in Nozick's (1974) experience machine, but this time not choosing to live in it for pleasure but for comfort. There is some evidence that people who commit violence that they have subsequently to disavow are not living in the 'real' world but in a dissociated state. It would follow from my earlier Spinozan requirement that spiritual well-being requires a grasp of reality in that a person cannot commit violence or harm to others and retain their spiritual well-being unless they are open to the full consequences for others of what they have done.

Strangely, people who are thoroughly bad in the larger world may inspire considerable loyalty in their family. Thus, it may be that empathy can be maintained for people with whom we have an interbrain connection – that is, those who are close to us and with whom we have a face-to-face relationship – even when there is no evidence that it is demonstrated in relation to strangers, even when that larger world believes that the person is a kind of monster.

Spirituality 101

In Chapter 2, Lord Layard was quoted as citing Jeremy Bentham's formula for happiness. It was a simple one – make someone else happy, and you will be happy yourself.

Auguste Comte, a convinced Darwinist, coined the term positivism. He argued that evolution applied to culture as well as to biology and assumed, contrary to Darwin, that evolution was directed in time towards better and better adaptation. There is no reason, of course, to suppose this. Only that evolution is a device for enabling organisms to make the most use of a constantly changing environment. Comte however saw progress in it and imposed this idea on spirituality. He thought that humankind, when first noting exceptional events that seemed to require an explanation, attributed them to gods. So the flood in the river was the river spirit being angry or weeping. As culture evolved, the next kind of explanation was metaphysical. The solar system was, for example, supposed to be a wonderful series of circular orbits as the celestial bodies swung round the earth in what the ancients thought was the most perfect figure. Eventually, as Comte saw it, human beliefs evolved to a third, advanced and rational stage, when the true explanation for floods, lightning and pestilence became apparent. They were caused by something and not intended by someone. This was the stage at which science was able to make the first positive contribution to knowledge.

Comte's positivism was opposed by many who thought, rightly, that he was an atheist. His atheism did not exclude spirituality and he invented a new, atheistic cult whose members worshipped and conducted services.

Positivism has been revived more recently as a synonym of empiricism, or the idea that we can only be sure of what we can sense. In this sense, positivism has become the preferred term of abuse in the social sciences for those who conduct quantitative research. There is, it is true, something anomalous about the conduct of much social science research in that, like technology, it sets out to find answers and solutions, bypassing the stage of ignorant but industrious curiosity that makes great physical scientists such appealing figures.

With the benefit of hindsight, one can see that Comte's view was very much a product of the European Enlightenment. He thought that people, or at least Europeans, were becoming more and more rational, and therefore better, and that this made them superior to those human beings who were less developed and to other animals who were lesser creations. But he also wanted to explain how this development was driven. He rejected a theistic explanation, so he could not posit a God who had created uniquely in human beings the ability to glimpse godhead and the means to strive towards it. Comte's alternative explanation was that it was society that created the glimpse of perfection that drove forwards rationalism. He thought that an individual human being did not just live for her- or himself but for, and through, others: 'pour autrui' (he wrote in French). This was translated into English as altruism, and it has had an almost universally bad press in recent years.

Sartre in particular singled out living 'pour autrui' as a kind of bad faith (Sartre, 1969). Instead of finding their own way, and exercising their own freedom, Sartre thought that people avoided facing up to their awareness of their own nothingness by assuming that they should do what others expected of them.

Sartre's focus was on consciousness although, rather confusingly, he called this *être* or being. His language is technical because he wanted to avoid other people's terms that he thought introduced error, but I will risk this and give an approximation of what he thought (Tantam, 2009 is a more detailed attempt to recreate Sartre's ideas). I will call the kind of consciousness that he called *être pour soi*, 'imagination'. Our imaginations contain nothing in themselves, but we can use them to imagine almost anything we choose. People generally only imagine things that are inside their experience, or calming or appropriate to their station in life, and this is true, Sartre thought, of what people imagine themselves to be – a consciousness that he called *être en soi*. People might also not want to imagine anything that would shock or upset others, or make anyone else think that they are bad or shameful. Thus, what people imagine about themselves might also be limited by other people's possible reactions and so their being is also constrained by social influences, which Sartre called *être pour autrui*. Sartre wanted to set his imagination free and not be limited in these ways. Free does not mean being, or doing, what we want, although Sartre's critics thought that it did. Sartre seemed to give himself considerable licence to do what he wanted in his private life, irrespective of his impact on other people, and this led these same critics to consider that both his life and his work were expressions of immorality. But this, in my view, underestimates the value of his ideas.

Our brief consideration of the basis of spirituality seems to have led us into an impasse. Everyone recognizes that people act cooperatively, that mothers look after babies, sometimes being willing to court extreme danger to protect them, and that we feel for other people. But this could all be explained without thinking that this connection takes us outside of ourselves at all. Mothers could be driven by a biological imperative – driven by oxytocin or vasopressin, some people might say – that has evolved because mothers whose genes encode this imperative have been more successful at conserving those genes in their babies. Or it may be that selflessness is really quite selfish. We look after our children because it is rewarding for us to do so (again, oxytocin might come into it) or perhaps we calculate that we will need to rely on them when we are older. Hume remarked on the fact that it was easier to empathize with someone similar to oneself, perhaps because it was easier to imagine oneself in the same circumstances, when one might then look for the same understanding from someone else.

Hume did not actually think that showing empathy (or sympathy as he called it) for someone else was actually a calculated deposit into the favour bank. He thought that it was pre-intellectual, an instinct that is embedded in human nature. Husserl called this 'intersubjectivity' arguing that other people's experience can under some circumstances be directly known to us. That may seem counter-intuitive, although many of us will have experiences that back this up. Sometimes these will be experiences of synchronicity. We may, for example, turn to someone we are with and start to comment on something, just as they turn to us and start their own comment. (Synchronicity does not always involve co-presence, but we need to invoke a more complex explanation than we give here – for further details, see Tantam, 2009.) At other times, we may glance across a room to our partner just as they look up at us, or we may find ourselves feeling caught up in a feeling of community or comradeship when we sing together or march in step.

Let's assume that mind and consciousness are the same (so we are excluding from this definition many of the automatic computational actions that the brain executes that would normally be considered mental activity), and that consciousness is what we can talk about to ourselves, i.e. what Vygotsky called 'inner language' (Vygotsky, 1966), or a flow of imagery that we can move about in the mind's eye, or sounds and music that we can imitate or hum. Consciousness is, as Sartre noted, self-serving. Using any of these types of imagery, language or music, we can imaginatively reconstruct the inner talk, imagery or hums of someone else – put ourselves in their shoes, as the saying goes, if we know them well enough. This ability is sometimes called 'theory of mind' because it originated as an observation about primates who unexpectedly seemed to guess at what conspecifics had experienced, even if they had not. Since it had been assumed that animals could not have a mind, this was a surprise, so researchers called the ability 'having a theory of mind'. Animals, including people, may also react with sadness or grief at the plight of other animals. Nowadays, this is often called 'cognitive empathy': cognitive, because it requires us to imagine what the other animal or person feels.

Sharing language or imagery with other people is a bit like sharing a house. It creates a closeness and various joint responsibilities and enjoyments. None of these would normally be described as a spiritual feeling, although they may be a source of well-being. The sharing is circumscribed by our mind but it does not go beyond it. It may lead to an intuition, apparently from nowhere, and this may be associated with a sense of relief or exhilaration similar to that when we are struck by a rhyme in a poem or a reference to another film in a film (Penrose, 1999: 543 gives a number of them), but these reinforce our sense of having a unique consciousness. They make us feel in the secret, not overawed by a secret that we can never grasp. The mystery of spirituality is not therefore provided by our minds, although we can and do imagine supernatural beings and, having an intuition of the mystery, we can invest it with symbols and music and ritual, all through conscious effort. The mystery is, counter-intuitively, provided by our brains. These are the bits of us that are connected up to other people, through a network of nonverbal communication. Our minds do not know what our brains are doing except through our observations of ourselves. So we are not directly aware of these reflexive communications, or of when our facial expressions mirror those of other people or our gaze switches to follow another person's gaze direction.

Not only does this 'interbrain' connection provide us with the spiritual intuition that each human being is connected to every other (and indeed to those animals who also follow our gaze and who experience emotional contagion to and from us), but it provides the basis for 'affective empathy', which means that we have immediate access to the emotions of other people through mirrored facial expression, leading to similar brain states in the people who are mirroring, and therefore to shared emotions. As we know, it is easy to turn off this kind of empathy (avoiding looking at another person's eyes is one way to do it) so we can take ourselves out of this connectedness, and indeed it may have been necessary for the development of an independent unshared mind in each individual that we did break the affective empathy connection. But the experience of full connection – often at times of particular mirroring like marching or singing together – lingers on to give us our sense of the transcendental.

Stillness

What practical applications do these rather abstract theories have? One direct one is that mental preoccupations drown out our appreciation of our interbrain connectedness. Hence the heading for this section is Stillness, a word taken from the Western interest in Zen and Japanese meditation practices that preceded the impact of a generation of Indian gurus. Meditation techniques are designed to achieve stillness and overcome mental distraction, by emptying our consciousness of content ('mindlessness'), by misdirecting our consciousness into something repetitive and therefore effortful but not absorbing (meditation using a mantra or cutting a lawn with scissors – the latter being a spiritual exercise once given to Christian nuns) or by focusing our attention on bodily sensation (and therefore on our brains too) and away from action, as in mindfulness meditation (Williams, 2010) or 'flow' experiences such as playing a musical instrument well or getting caught up in a sport.

Meditation does, as my hypothesis predicts, increase empathy (Lesh, 1970a, 1970b; Newman, 1994) and one's sense of social connectedness (Hutcherson et al., 2008). However, these studies did not include a control group and it may be that any intervention that requires people to pause and take time out of a busy day will reduce anxiety non-specifically, whether the intervention is relaxation, yoga (Sharma et al., 2008) or just having a nap. When a control group is included, it seems to be the self-control elements of meditation that exceed the effects of the control interventions (Smith, 1976).

It is a lot easier to learn mindfulness meditation than it is to play the violin well, and mindfulness has had much greater impact than music therapy as a spiritual intervention. Mindfulness meditation has been incorporated into the currently very popular cognitive behavioural therapy (CBT) as an extension of the schema-based therapy approach that tried to disclose the assumptions that colour our thoughts rather than simply focusing on our thoughts or cognitions as they influence mood. It was a measure to improve autobiographical memory – impaired in depression – and therefore a treatment to prevent the recurrence of depression, for which it was shown to be effective (Teasdale et al., 2000). However, it was then found to enhance well-being even in the absence of depression, both by increasing positive feelings and reducing negative ones (Keng et al., 2011).

These effects have been anecdotally claimed for other meditative and other flow practices, too, and we will not therefore assume that they are limited to mindfulness meditation.

Meditation produces characteristic EEG slowing and fMRI changes (Cahn & Polich, 2006) that point to a redistribution of neural activity during meditation, although the function of the network that becomes more active is unclear. Experienced meditators are less likely to shift into the default network (Brewer et al., 2011). The default network is active in day-dreaming, dreaming and thinking about the past. Day-dreaming about people we are close to increases our sense of connectedness to them, and so enhances life satisfaction, but day-dreaming about strangers increases our sense of loneliness (Mar et al., 2012). It has been suggested that it involves recalling memories and refreshing the emotions with which they have been tagged, an exercise which, if it occurs deliberately, we would call nostalgia (Hepper et al., 2012). Interestingly, nostalgia increases not just our connectedness with our pasts but our sense of being connected to others (Batcho, 2007), suggesting that long-term meditation may increase self-control but at the expense of social connectedness. One possible reason for this inconsistency may be that the effects of regular meditation are contrary to the effects of new or occasional meditation (Crane et al., 2010). This would be consistent with the emotional detachment from human relationships that many regular meditators develop.

Most of the time, our consciousness focuses instrumentally on what we can do with or for nature, or with or for people. The interbrain, or the connectedness, that is linked to well-being is not instrumental, not as Buber (1958) has it, I–it, but I–thou. Even in nature, when we connect to it, we feel it to be alive and capable of pain or happiness depending on how we react to it. Connectedness with nature (Cervinka et al., 2012), with the universe, with humanity or a social institution and with the universe or Gaia – all of these seem to have a similar effect. We would argue that connectedness or interbrain bandwidth is a disposition that spans each of these domains, so that someone who becomes more attentive to their natural surroundings also becomes more attentive to other people as 'subjects' in their own world.

The here and now

Spiritual guides often focus on the present moment, perhaps aware that people who live in the past are often trying to change it and people who live in the future are often trying to manipulate it. Both of these efforts are avoidance of the real, in the same sense that Nozick's (1974) experience machine is, since they are driven by an urge to make life over according to a personal formula, rather than to live it as given. Living in the past or future also means that one is only half alive in the present. Dr Seuss wrote, or possibly Gabriel Lorca, or possibly it is just a proverb that echoes Aristippus whose hedonism I introduced in the first chapter, 'Don't cry because it's over, smile because it happened'.

Every moment that we want to get over as soon as possible, or that we would rather pretend was not happening, is a moment lost from life. So the total span of fully lived life is reduced. One of the first philosophers to formulate this was Nietzsche, who, in several places, proposed that although we have the perception of living from moment to moment, each moment may 'eternally recur' if we are fated to live and re-live our lives. In *The Gay Science* (1882/2001), he imagined a demon telling the reader that this was to happen and that

> every pain and every joy and every thought and sigh and everything unutterably small or great in your life will have to return to you, all in the same succession and sequence – even this spider and this moonlight between the trees, and even this moment and I myself. (ibid., section 34)

The point of Nietzsche's thought experiment, for this is what it is, is to test whether or not the reader is 'well disposed' to themselves – in other words, if they have the greatest possible life satisfaction, for if they do they would, Nietzsche thought, '*crave nothing more fervently* than this ultimate eternal confirmation and seal'.

Engagement

Engagement with life is one characteristic of those who live long (Hutnik et al., 2012). Volunteering can provide both emotional engagement and social connectedness, and has been found to increase mental health, irrespective of cultural values (Pilkington et al., 2012). Spirituality may be associated with an intensification of present experience, perhaps through the here and now focus associated with spirituality. However, spiritual preoccupations may also increase at times of emotional crisis and these may either provoke withdrawal from engagement or an intensification of it. Withdrawal from engagement follows from the defeat that we considered in Chapter 3. One factor that counteracts defeat is that life has too much meaning to back off from it.

The meaning of life

Victor Frankl (1963) almost lost his 'will to live' (to use another term of Nietzsche's) in the concentration camp, but came even closer to losing it after the initial euphoria of liberation had passed and he discovered how many of his close family had died. It was his second wife who got him through. She was his typist at first, but she believed his simple but constantly reiterated message: one must live a life with meaning. Frankl himself seems to have found this meaning in nature, particularly in climbing, but it was obviously not enough to feel uplifted in the mountains. So his life, and his wife Ella's life too, gained meaning through his dedication to disseminating his message to other people, as a healing.

Many people would echo Frankl in thinking that a life without meaning, or purpose, is an empty life, hardly worth living. It is hardly better than living through the experience machine that we started this chapter by describing. Frankl's life, which was long by the standards of his generation, exemplifies the elements that we suggest constitute a life lived well: transcendent experience (climbing in Frankl's case); connectedness (Ventegodt et al., 2003), which, for Frankl, was provided by his writing, lecturing and the many contacts he made through his ideas; engagement (Frankl never seems to have been far from his Dictaphone, so that he could write down a new idea whenever during the day or night it occurred); and value to others. Frankl's value to others never seems to have been in doubt in his mind, because he was a healer.

The negative side of spirituality: terror

Sartre, a considerable sceptic about spirituality, imagined a political version that did not involve, as he thought that other spirituality did, one person coercing others. He thought of Parisians in the first days of revolution and how they began to act spontaneously but synchronously, and then as more or more restrictions were placed on them by the government, began to define themselves as a unity in 'negation' to the government so much so that their consciousness 'fused' into one group in which no one was a leader or a follower, but all were acting and feeling – a recognizably spiritual experience, provoked by the intense fear and excitement caused by the riot.

However, Sartre imagined what would happen in the future. He supposed that the sans-culottes would meet again to celebrate their success in throwing tyranny over, and would feel the same sense of togetherness and well-being. But at their next reunion, one of them might feel that they were a bit too busy to come, and the others would feel diminished, perhaps would pass a motion to insist on everyone attending or else. But what would be the 'or else'? Sartre thought that this was the origin of the phase of the revolution called the 'terror', and that it was terror that also maintained other groups in a fused state: terror at being deprived of closeness to others but also terror of what the group might do to defectors. So he supposed that spirituality has a negative as well as a positive side. This is reflected in many organized religions, which include terror about 'damnation', being consumed by Djinns or demons, and other terrifying punishments after death in their methods of encouraging the faithful to follow the correct path.

Ernest Becker (1973) proposed that people were motivated by a denial of death, and this led to a revival of Sartre's term or rather its English translation (Sartre's word was 'la terreur') in the formulation of 'terror management theory'. Kierkegaard, Heidegger and other existential philosophers, in numerous books and papers, have explored the importance of death anxiety, and of facing mortality in their own lives. Ernest Becker was interested in how people characteristically suppress their fear of death, both individually and in society. At the time of publication of his book, *The Denial of Death*, the Hero archetype of Jung had been used as the basis for a new personal spirituality in books by Joseph Campbell (2008) and others. It was influential because it provided a kind of rationale for the drug-fuelled introspections so characteristic of the 1960s and 1970s. Becker proposed a different reason for the popularity of this archetype: that the hero was portrayed as a kind of immortal, and that in identifying with a hero (much less often a heroine), readers of Joseph Campbell, Carlos Castaneda and others, could imagine that they, too, need not fear death.

Terror management theory assumes, like psychoanalysis, that it is the very fact that people do not think about death that confirms they are anxious about it. Evidence for this comes from speculation, but also from more empirical measures such as the content analysis of replies to questions about death and sentence completion tests in which people are asked to complete stems, like 'coff-'. If they complete this as 'coff-ee', there is no evidence of death anxiety, but if they complete this as 'coff-in', there is. Although terror management theory has stimulated a great deal of research, the effect size in studies is small and death anxiety is readily suppressed when asking people to be 'rational' (Simon et al., 1997). Death anxiety may be more of an issue for college students and Americans than other groups (Burke et al., 2010).

The approach of death is an important stimulant to spiritual thoughts, and a feeling of closeness to God (another kind of connectedness) and strong religious beliefs have been found in several studies to be associated with a reduction in distress and greater acceptance of death (Daaleman & Dobbs, 2010). Hence, death is not always denied or even feared. However, there is no doubt that when it is feared, it opens the door to unscrupulous religious figures and healers.

Spirituality, like every aspect of life, has a dark side. In the next chapter, the psychotherapist's viewpoint, we will consider the paradoxical idea that it is this very shadow that is essential for joy, just as the black pigment in a painting is essential to bringing out the white.

8

The Psychotherapist's Viewpoint

Suppose that Fred is one of our readers and that he has just got to this point in the book. He wants to be happy and healthy but in the right way, so he has been making some notes of what we have said about positive psychology, healthy living and spirituality. Today, feeling inspired by what he has read, he has decided that he will go for a long walk in nature and open himself up to its joys.

Two hours after he was due to set off, however, Fred is still at home. First of all, it was a bit too cool, and there was a threat of rain, so he thought it best not to set off immediately. Then he decided to have some extra toast if he was going to be active all day. Breakfast television pointed him to a feature film that he wanted to watch and that proved quite engrossing.

Four hours later, Fred is still at home, although feeling exhausted. He had hunted out his hiking boots, which had taken quite some time, and then he had needed to put waterproof stuff on them. He couldn't find the woolly hat that he knew he had somewhere, and particularly wanted to wear. Then he did not feel quite enough energy to do the full walk that he had planned (10 miles), so he had spent a long time working out a shorter, still circular route. This meant a lot of checking on what different map symbols meant. Eventually, Fred postponed his plans to the following weekend and decided to have a healthy lunch instead.

Fred's failure to act on his plans to do something healthy would be, according to Socrates, accounted for by ἀκρασία (akrasia), often translated, and noted in an earlier chapter, as weakness of will although actually meaning a lack of power (krasia is the ending of other kinds of power, like demokrasia – democracy or people power). Weakness of will fits with a particular, imperialist view of human nature that was popular in the Roman Empire and later in the UK, at the height of the British Empire, in the 19th century. It is still present in commonsense psychology, where it seems natural to attribute people's failings to uphold commitments to their lack of will power.

If a person knew that something was in their best interest, why would they need particular power to carry this through (Hare, 2001)? The answer, according to Donald Davidson (1980), is that we do not always turn decisions into actions. He called it 'continence', when we do. His explanation for Fred's backsliding would have been that he was 'incontinent'.

I have already considered a number of possible causes of incontinence. Defeat was one: defeated people give up on continence. Another possibility is that continence is effortful and requires the expenditure of a resource – possibly dopamine related – that can get depleted if it isn't replenished by reward (Baumeister et al., 1998). A persistent lack of reward might therefore lead to incontinence. Continence might also require external resources – for example, Fred might need access to transport to go for his walk – and these may be unreliable or absent. But perhaps the most likely explanation of incontinence is conflict. Terror management theorists and existentialists argue that one of the major conflicts in life is that we plan as if we will be there to carry out our plans, but in fact we might suddenly die and be unable to. We might make a rational decision about our chances, but many people make emotional decisions apparently based on the irrational belief that they are personally immortal. The 'hedonist immortals' described in Chapter 2, who may take in government warnings about over-eating or smoking but do not act on them, are incontinent because, so a terror management theorist would claim, they deal with the inevitability of death by pretending that it does not matter to them.

Unlike terror management theorists, rationalists assume that people are motivated by their own best interests, although they may be muddled or misled by faulty learning into pursuing interests that they believe are in their best interests but are not. The possibility of people having conflicting intentions, including some which are against their best interests, does not fit into this scheme. Incontinence is one example of such ambivalence. Otherwise, it would be possible to both intend to diet and intend to carry out the desire to eat that particularly delectable cake; or intend to take the tablets for blood pressure and then put off taking the prescription (Sripada, 2010). Possibly the most simple explanation of incontinence is that it can be attributed to conflicting intentions, values, motives or emotions. This is possibly the most commonly held view among non-psychologists: that someone is too mixed up to know what is best for them. Akrasia would be, on these accounts, about conflict.

Theories of conflict that have founded psychotherapy approaches

Psychoanalysis

Freud, along with his mentor Breuer, belonged to the Berlin Psychophysical Society, and was, like other members, committed to an energetic explanation of mental activity. He thought that the brain was like a machine that was driven by some energy or 'cathexis', possibly the newly discovered electrical force, and that by tracing the flow of this energy (which he called 'Q'), one could explain mental as well as brain processes. He described this in a work that was only published posthumously, *The Project for a Scientific Understanding of Psychology* (Bilder & LeFever, 1998). Q was created, Freud supposed, autochthonously by φ neurons. Q had to be transferred to motor, ψ, neurons to be discharged, but there was a barrier between the two neurons. The barrier could be overcome by ω neurons that were activated by organs of special sense. So when we see something that needs action, Freud supposed that ω neurons are activated and they allow cathexis to flow into ψ neurons from Φ neurons and so have the energy to activate effectors, such as muscles. Later, Freud substituted psychic 'structures' for neuronal populations; Φ neurons became the unconscious and later the Id; Ψ neurons became the ego. The barrier between the two became a psychological function, 'repression'. Cathexis turned from an actual energy created by nerve cell metabolism into a psychological energy or drive, the libido, created by a wish for stimulation of sensory receptors in the sexual areas: the whole skin in the infant, and the genitals post-puberty. We need this barrier, Freud thought, to stop us from behaving like animals, who Freud supposed would be constantly in a rut did they not have an oestrous cycle to bridle them.

All of us are therefore, in the eyes of the Freudian psychoanalyst, constantly in conflict over how to allow sexual desire to find a direct outlet in sexual activity. Civilization, Freud believed, requires that sexual impulses – or indeed other impulses – are not immediately acted on, hence the need for repression. But this raises the issue of what to do with the energy that has not found its expression.

There have been many modifications of psychoanalytic theory, but all of them contain a theory of unconscious drives or yearnings, a theory that these drives or yearnings may be opposed or frustrated by other people, and the presumption that how we deal with a frustrated drive or yearning determines our mental health. Attachment theory, a development of psychoanalysis, presumes that the energizer of action is the desire to be close to a mother figure when a threat creates anxiety. This is in many ways a very different formulation to that of Freud, not least because anxiety comes before the desire for closeness, whereas in Freud's model it is a consequence of the barrier against the impulse-finding expression. However, attachment theory follows the same basic pattern, in supposing that the wrong kind of mothering fails to make the infant secure. Either this leads to a tendency to become over-preoccupied with security, taking away from the freedom and energy directed towards other goals and leading to an increase in negative feelings; or it leads to a dampening down of anxiety responses, along with other emotional responding, at least in adulthood (Adam et al., 2004). Reduced positive and increased negative feelings independently lead to a reduction in well-being, as we have noted in previous chapters.

Psychoanalysts have contributed many case studies and anecdotes that provide evidence that people are diverted into acts that seem to undermine their own plans. These include the symptoms that Freud called hysterical or obsessional; intensive preoccupations with sexual activities that are, as Freud said, not directed towards reproduction; a series of failed relationships that seem to repeat the same pattern over and over; and more trivial but undermining experiences, such as memory lapses, lost objects, unaccountable resentments and angry outbursts.

Existential psychotherapy

Existential psychotherapy originates in philosophy, and in particular in the philosophy of being. It supposes that being self-aware creates anxieties because we can imagine a world without limit, and yet we are always faced with what Jaspers called 'limit situations' (Jaspers, 1956). One of these is the one that terror management theorists have also focused on – the inevitability of death. Another is that of never being able to be as close to another person as we are to ourselves. The conflict is how much to allow ourselves to be aware of the anxieties that are fundamental to being who we are – 'ontological' is the term often used – and how much to throw ourselves into automatic pilot and live from day to day without thinking of how much time we have left or how little basis we have for thinking that we can predict how other people will react in the future. Throwing ourselves completely into ordinary life implies a degree of self-deception and, like any other deception, this often creates anxiety about being caught out. Hence, at least some of our motivation gets diverted from carrying out our current plans into sustaining our self-deceptions.

Schema theory

Nisbett and colleagues (Nisbett et al., 1973) changed the direction of cognitive psychology by introducing the notion of cognitive schemata. Rather than thoughts being created by observations, we have pre-existing schemata, partly developed from prior observations, which we place over our sensory world in the process of being aware of it. Some of these schemata, cognitive therapists maintain, are influenced by desired experience rather than actual experience. Thus, effort has to be directed either into altering experience to fit the pre-existing schema better (which may mean choosing sub-optimal experiences) or into altering experience during processing in order to avoid having to change the schema. There is a conflict between maintaining the schema and cleaving to a more accurate perception of reality. Both entail disequilibrium, but changing the schema possibly more so.

Trauma theory

Psychological traumata are, by definition, highly emotionally coloured experiences that cannot be processed and encoded into long-term memory. They interfere with the memorization of subsequent experiences, and cause avoidance of new experiences that may re-evoke the trauma. The conflict here is between the past experience and the current one. Previous trauma is associated with increased rates of depression, anxiety and substance misuse, all of which have negative effects on well-being.

There is a further possible conflict in trauma, which is that people who have experienced a trauma want to change the past. It is possible to change appraisals of the past: for example, saying to oneself, it's over now, gone and time to move on. But this is not what traumatized people want. They want the past to be different. Once again, there is a conflict, this time between what a person wishes for and what is likely to happen.

Predicaments

Predicaments are situations in which a person is faced with several possible choices but cannot resolve them. Predicaments may be created by any of the conflict theories we have just discussed, or may simply result from the motivational conflict of wanting to make both, or neither, of the choices.

It will be apparent that the very different psychotherapy theories that we have reviewed (and, in fact, almost all psychotherapy theories) make two presumptions:

Presumption 1: Conflict is as much a part of our inner as our outer life

None of us is likely to be fully 'continent' in the sense of being fully able to realize our well-being. However, the more aware we are of our conflicts, the more likely we are to minimize this lack of continence. Mahatma Gandhi captured this when he wrote: 'Happiness is when what you think, what you say, and what you do are in harmony.' (cited in Michelli, 1988: 88)

Presumption 2: Negative feelings are normal

Negative feelings play an important role in life and are not to be avoided. Anxiety is, as Freud (Laplanche, 1988) noted, a signal of conflict as well as danger or threat. We need it to alert us to a situation that needs attention and resolution. A lack of anxiety feelings might mean that someone is unconflicted, but may also mean that the person is not sufficiently monitoring danger in their environment (Lohr, 2012; Robinson et al., 2012). Anxiety is a normal, and protective, emotion. Anxiety should not be avoided or minimized but used. Anger, depression and even jealousy have important roles to play, as Emmy van Deurzen has extensively documented (Van Deurzen, 2009). We recognize this in the case of shame since to be shameless is to be a potential risk to other people.

Our negative feelings also make us more sensitive to the feelings of others.

Ego

Freud's Project (Levy, 2002) developed out of an assumption that brain and mind were intimately connected, but, as we have already noted, he then switched emphasis from a theory of mind to a theory of 'Ich' or ego development. 'Ich' he defined to be that bit of our mind that we are aware of, what we think of as who we are but also what we know about ourselves that others cannot know. It is closely related to what other psychotherapists call 'self': the entity apparently referred to in the adage, 'Physician, know thyself'. Of course, 'know thyself' is a reflexive expression with self playing the part of 'here' in 'come here' or 'now' in 'do it now'. Freud's 'Ich' refers both to the 'I' and the 'myself' in 'I do know myself'. These are, as Gilbert Ryle (Ryle, 2009) might say, 'category errors'. There is an apocryphal story that when Carl Rogers was asked to define 'self', he said that he had a patient who would answer a question from Dr Rogers along the lines of 'how are you feeling in your-self today?' or 'how do you deal with that yourself?' by answering: 'My self is fine, thank you, doctor' or 'My self seems lost and does not know what to do'. After a while, Rogers got into the habit of asking this patient about his self, and not himself.

The reason that there are theories of ego or self-development is not that Freud or Rogers were dumb, but that they addressed what we all believe about ourselves – that we have a part of us that only we know, that speculates, thinks, waits, plans, wants, loves, and so on. These are all activities that go beyond the immediate challenges of a situation into areas of which we can have no direct knowledge, an ability that Brentano (1973), one of Freud's lecturers, considered to be the *sine qua non* of mind, its intentionality or grasp.

When a good friend tells us that they are unhappy, we ask 'why?': in other words, what have they been keeping quiet about, what have they been speculating about, what have they been grieving over that might explain being unhappy? We are asking them to, as Freud might say, reveal the contents of their ego (Meeks & Jeste, 2009).

Freud's model of the mind and its conflicts was memorably pilloried in a lecture that I attended, where the speaker said the image that Freud's theory of the unconscious brought to his mind was of a timid bank manager (the ego) refereeing a fight between a maiden aunt (the super-ego) and a sex-crazed gorilla (the id). A more up to date anal-ogy might be of a boardroom with no people present but plans in the place of directors. Each plan has its own emotions, values and action schemas attached, and competes for resources (Huang & Bargh, to be published), whilst the arbitrating chief executive (it is supposed that the mind or brain has an 'executive' function) gives the go-ahead to the winning plan. The upshot of this model of conflict is not dissimilar to Freud's: if the executive cannot decide on one clear course of action, or if two conflicting plans each get partly supported, the organization functions less effectively.

'Control yourself', 'master your desires', 'take control of your life' are appeals that people still make to each other's wills but on the boardroom analogy they should be getting their plans to interact, negotiating between them as it were, and putting the needs of the whole organization/organism first over each particular plan. The chief executive is more likely to give the go-ahead to collaborating plans. Neuroscientists have identified a part of the brain, in the prefrontal cortex, that seems to be most active during motivational conflicts, in an area that is often associated with executive function and sometimes even with 'the will' (suppos-ing that there is one) (Meeks & Jeste, 2009). So perhaps there is some backing to this new metaphor. However, it is somewhat dry as dust. No doubt boardroom arguments can become quite heated, but few people would join a board of directors to experience the full range of emotions that life can provide. Plans are just one aspect of how people choose their futures. Passions and impulses, even hopeless, stupid or self-destructive ones, come into it too.

Alternative explanations of akrasia

In its customary usage, akrasia means failing to impose self-control or self-regulation, even when this is going to be manifestly advantageous in the long run. Our experience of akrasia is often something along the lines of 'I can't be bothered' or 'it's too much of a hassle'. The 'I' in these statements is lacking whatever is needed to deal with, bother with or keep on target with in the case of a hassle. We sometimes feel the depletion as an actual lack of something. In Chapter 1, I termed this 'reward' and mentioned research (Wagner et al., 2013) that strongly indicates that the neurochemical equivalent of this reward is a lack of activity in dopaminergic neurones in the nucleus accumbens. Thus, one simple explanation for akrasia is that it is due to a physiological state, sometimes simplified into a 'lack of dopamine'. There is some evidence for this in people with ADHD, which is associated with reduced dopamine efferent effects on the frontal lobes, and in people with a cocaine habit who are in withdrawal.

We are only too aware that people are very different when it comes to finding a route to happiness. Although people rarely appeal to will power these days, concepts like self-control and emotional regulation figure in today's psychological research and this research demonstrates that many people find that increasing their emotional regulation and self-control increases their happiness and well-being. Analysis of a 32-year follow-up of 1000 children (Moffitt et al., 2011) led the authors to conclude that 'childhood self-control predicts physical health, substance dependence, personal finances, and criminal offending outcomes' and that 'interventions addressing self-control might reduce a panoply of societal costs, save taxpayers money, and promote prosperity' (2011: 2693).

One problem with both the science and commonsense psychology of this is that they fit into a mindset that in the political sphere would be called colonialist. This mindset is reinforced by an assumption that the mind and the brain are very closely related. So the part of the brain that has expanded most in human beings compared to other apes, and that has most expanded in apes compared to other mammals (the prefrontal cortex), is the part that is also assumed to have this executive or self-control function. The prefrontal cortex has many connections with other parts of the brain, and has an inhibitory effect on many of them, and this makes it the head office, but it could just be the equivalent of the receptionist, taking lots of calls and turning lots of them away, but putting some through to any of the other departments with which it is connected.

Will, too, seems like a colonialist idea. Why would the mind be organized like an empire, or like an organization with a chief executive, any more than the brain? Tolstoy, in *War and Peace* (Tolstoy, 2010), famously put forward a completely different conception of will in his portrayal of Field Marshall Kutusov, in charge of the Russian forces defending Russia from Napoleon's invasion. Kutusov blocked all of the actions of his officers who wanted to attack. He kept retreating, even allowing Moscow to be taken and burnt, leaving the Russian winter, and Napoleon's over-extended supply lines, to defeat the French. One possible function of 'will' might therefore be, on analogy with this, to inhibit rapid and immediate actions, as the self-regulation model indeed suggests. It might be like a committee that never takes action until it is over-ridden by someone taking an unconstitutional action.

Tolstoy thought that even the degree of individual power that we have just described over-estimated Kutusov's influence. He thought that the Russian army itself somehow knew what to do and, in a shambolic way, did it.

Non-conflictual approaches to incontinence

This brings us to a completely different way of looking at the will (or 'ego' or 'the self'). The two approaches that we will consider are sometimes called the 'narrative approach' and the 'dramaturgical approach'.

The narrative approach

Let's consider this situation. Enid is laying the table. Her husband, Alf, comes in and starts to fuss with the place settings. Enid says, 'What's wrong? I'm doing it fine, aren't I?' Alf says, 'What's your problem, I'm only trying to help'. Enid says, 'Nothing I do is ever good enough for you'. Alf says, 'Here we go again. Why can't you just accept that I have more idea of proper manners than you do?' Enid at that point knocks over a glass, which breaks. Alf says, 'Hey, you've just smashed my favourite glass. You did that on purpose'. Enid says, 'I'm sorry, it was an accident. I didn't choose it. I was just so upset. You know I can be a bit clumsy when I'm upset'. Alf says, 'You should learn to control yourself better'.

Nowadays, we might be unwilling to accept that Alf was right to blame Enid's lack of self-control. There definitely feels like some bullying going on that is likely to have made anyone anxious and therefore clumsy. Many researchers would now consider that many actions we take do not allow for conscious reflection because thinking about things takes time, often too much time. So we would be inclined to think that Enid's account, thinking of the glass as a bit of Alf, was something that she thought up afterwards to explain what happened. I have previously pointed out (Tantam & Mace, 1999) that people sometimes use 'because' to mean what caused me to do something, but sometimes it means, 'here is my justification for why I did this'. For example, if I say that I was late 'because' I went to bed late, that might be true but it might also be true that I would never be late getting up to watch the omnibus of *EastEnders* even if I had been to bed late. So I might be offering an excuse for my lack of control over my time-keeping, in which case it would be an act of incontinence. Enid is making the opposite kind of excuse: she was not intending anything – it was 'an accident' and no will or intention was involved.

We might accept Enid's idea that she did not do it on purpose. It is rare for people to deliberately break something unless they do so in an obvious and dramatic way. But let's say Enid's therapist, when discussing the whole episode, reminded Enid it was Alf's favourite glass, and Enid said, 'Well, I wasn't really choosing his glass, but when I look back I might have picked up the glass more roughly than usual because it was like a bit of Alf'. Or, she might have said, 'I just hated that glass. Every time I did something with it, I was a bit rough with it. I guess I was even rougher that time'.

Enid said that she had got into a habit of roughly handling that particular glass. Habits influence our actions very quickly. Hence, it is quite plausible that Enid's clumsiness, her anxiety and her habit of treating that particular glass roughly did come together to cause her to break it, and even that at some time in the future a group of neurones associated with the habit of handling roughly would be shown to be active when Enid sighted that particular glass, and that this activation preceded the firing of the motor neurons associated with knocking the glass over. She might even say that this habit was one of the 'reasons' that she broke the glass, meaning that it caused her to break the glass. If this were true, she could say that she was not responsible for wanting to hurt Alf.

Her therapist encouraged Enid to talk the incident through, and, in the process, Enid came to some conclusions about herself. She might have formulated them to herself in different ways. She might have said, for example, 'I hadn't realized how much I want to hurt Alf for all the hurt he has done me' or she might have said, 'I really worry that I am so afraid of Alf that I take it out on an innocent glass' or 'I thought that I was rather an empty person, but now I realize I'm having a lot more emotions than I realized'.

Narrative theorists would say that all of these comments that Enid makes to herself about herself contribute to what makes up her 'self' or her ego. (As it happens, this is also consistent with the prefrontal cortex-as-executive model of brain function, since the evidence points to this area of the brain as being crucial to narrative.) This inner narrative idea was first put forward by Vygotsky (1966), who thought of it as the core of consciousness. It's one explanation for why people talk to themselves, for talking to yourself out loud is one way of strengthening the narrative when one is doing a tricky job and trying not to make a mistake, or when one is pushing oneself to do something difficult.

Ricœur (1984) was one of the first psychologically minded philosophers to put forward a narrative approach to identity, but the idea has found favour with sociologists (Giddens, 1991) and psychologists (Singer et al., 2012). Commentaries on the world might also take the form of images or sounds associated with experience or reflection, but for simplicity we will focus on talk to or about the self. Of course, much self-talk is transitory: muttering to oneself in the supermarket, 'Don't forget the eggs' does not amount to a core statement about who or what we are. However, thinking sadly 'I would have dearly loved to be a dancer' obviously belongs in a story about oneself. One difference between the two statements is that the second includes a value, 'dearly loved', that tags the importance of the statement and an emotion word that tags the contribution of this fragment of self-narrative to health – in this case, a negative one.

To make this a full theory of self, we need to add two further elements. One is an aspiration or aim, as in wanting to be a dancer, and the other is memory. We need to recall previous narratives and to haul in episodes from our autobiographical memory. So, if Alf were to want to make it up to Enid, and asked her if she would like a weekend away, she would want to think this over. Thinking it over would involve talking to herself (and perhaps talking to Alf) in which she evokes previous conversations, fragments of magazine stories, conversations with her mother about weekends away or daydreams of her own about it. Each of these fragments about weekends away is likely to evoke a memory, usually an image or a sound or a smell, coupled with an emotion. Evoking and processing these would lead to Enid's answer: that is, if her imagery did not get overwhelmed by images of Alf when he is thwarted or on holiday.

Self-talk is only one kind of talk, and a great deal of other talk too is about identity. Even in this conversation between Alf and Enid, he is likely to make assertions about Enid's preferences since he is almost bound to say, at some point, 'Come on, I know you'll love it when we get there'. Enid's self-talk also brings in other narratives itself: what her mother said, what people write in magazines about weekends away or about giving your husband a second chance, an advertisement that she might have seen about weekend breaks. Some of these fragments may well have turned into values in Enid's memory: that she deserves some time off, for example, or that she is always one to give a person a second chance.

We can see how the narrative account fits well with Aristotle's ideas about eudaimonia. He thought that each time we make a choice we should plan to act ahead of time in a way that increases our long-term well-being rather than our short-term gratification. This is what Enid is trying to do in our illustration. Very often, though, we do not have time to make a conscious choice and we rely on habit. Alf may have come home and said, 'come on Enid, I've booked us into a hotel. We've got to leave in 15 minutes'. Enid would have had to act on instinct. Out of the habit of compliance, she might go. But then she would reflect on her decision after, as she did on breaking Alf's glass, and this may have led her either to confirm that she did the right thing, in which case she would hesitate less in future, or to become determined that, in future, she was not going to go along with Alf's rash decisions. Reflection afterwards on a choice can change the emotional flavour of the choice we made, and perhaps also of the choice we did not. So Enid may revive the memory of when she first heard Alf come out with the weekend away, and make it much more negative, whilst the choice to stay at home would gain a much more positive emotional flavour. The same process of re-evaluation of an impulse decision – to have a stiff drink after a really bad day at work, perhaps – might reduce our likelihood of doing that in future rather than, say, going for an evening walk. These small decisions add up, when taken together, to strong tendencies towards processing negative feelings and choosing suppression instead. Since suppression leads to greater fatigue from work, using suppression less is likely to improve health (van Gelderen et al., 2011). Emotional suppression may also have a negative impact on relationships. If one member of a couple suppresses his or her grief over a bereavement, in order to spare the other partner's feelings, both partners will have a more negative reaction to the bereavement in the long run (Stroebe et al., 2013).

The dramaturgical approach

We have considered narrative mediated by self-talk, but the first exposure to tales for most of us is the stories that are told to us by other people. These stories may start very early on in life. So self-narratives are really those told by us but also to us, about ourselves. Ernaux (2008) used this sentiment, that she attributed to José Ortega y Gasset, as an epigraph in the preface to her novel, *Les Années*: 'Nous n'avons que notre histoire, et elle n'est pas à nous' (We only have our story, and it does not belong to us). These stories are emotive, as well as descriptive. People close to us can make us hate ourselves, or love ourselves as well as know ourselves, or be deceived about ourselves.

An alternative metaphor for how we come to think of ourselves is dramaturgical – that we are more like characters in a play about ourselves. Many of the words that we use for our and other people's natures are taken from drama – personality, character, role, part, script, actor and person itself.

The inner narrative is like an aside in a play, one that the other characters do not hear. There is no particular reason to consider therefore that the aside comes first – a playwright might choose to have their principal character address the audience before the play proper begins, or may omit asides altogether, and there is no reason to assume that what Freud called ego develops before the infant knows about the world around them. Nor is there any particular reason to privilege descriptions of what goes on inside people's heads, or rather what is going on of which they are aware over what they are actually saying to other people. This is reflected even in psychoanalysis in its relational turn (Beebe, 2003). It is more fully developed in existential psychotherapy, which is rooted in Heidegger's concept of 'existence' (Dasein) or 'self and others in relation'.

Interpersonal conflict

Goffman (1997) drew his metaphor for akrasia from the theatre. His 'dramaturgical' model was based on the difference in people's behaviour in social settings, or 'on the stage' or 'behind the scenes'. At times, he seems deeply suspicious of other people's power to harm: another theoretical contribution was 'stigma', which considered how identity could be 'spoiled' by other people (Goffman, 1963). Being on stage required 'face work' (Goffman, 1969) to prevent the performance breaking down, and meant that people were always to some degree pretending to be what they were not. The tension between being what others expected and fulfilling one's own goals could lead to akrasia if our personal goals would not be socially approved. Sartre came to the same conclusion in *Being and Nothingness*, as expressed in his concept of 'mauvaise foi' or bad faith (Sartre, 1969).

Social conformity may be a factor in suppressing antisocial or impulsive behaviour and may thus increase life satisfaction in the long run, but that assumes that the society to which one is conforming has the interests of the individual at heart. Having offenders in the family increases the risk of offending when children grow up (Farrington, 1995) and is one likely explanation that a good 'performance' in life allows for offending.

Although I have used the metaphor of narrative to depict the dynamic interchange of our thoughts about ourselves, and our plans and intentions, and our conversations with other people, Goffman's metaphor of the theatre is probably closer to the truth. 'Narrative' in this psychological sense is not purely verbal. It includes symbols and signs. In fact, it is more like seeing an actual performance of a play, and therefore experiencing how the actors dress, how they speak their lines, the setting and all the other things that we might remember more than the lines, than simply reading the play. More than that, what we remember of the play is different again from our contemporaneous experience of watching it. Ego, or self, or inner narrative: all of these ideas include memory as well as current awareness. Emotion colours and indexes these memories according to, what I have called, the emotional flavour of the lived experience (Tantam, 2003). Emotional indexing of this kind is receiving increasing support from the field of neuroscience (Bossert et al., 2011; Eskine et al., 2011; Whissell, 1991).

Goffman's dramaturgical model makes the potential conflict in human relationships central. It is easy to assume that relationships are always positive. Social contact with other people is often termed 'social support' on the supposition that the more contact the better. Similarly, it is often assumed that having close relationships is always good for everyone. I have referred to the evidence for this in previous chapters. The evidence is often associational (Barger et al., 2009) and, as such, can go both ways. Well-being may increase the likelihood of having close relationships as well as be increased by them. Longitudinal studies paint a rather more complex picture. In one study that followed a cohort of adolescents into middle age, only peer rejection in adolescence predicted life satisfaction in middle age, but that was only in those who did not have friends in adolescence. Having friends protected against, or so the authors concluded, this negative effect of relationships (Khor et al., 2014). There is a trend at the moment to attribute these negative effects to having relationships with people who have a 'dark side' (Ali & Chamorro-Premuzic, 2010). Conflicts in intimate relationships are often attributed to the other person's 'psychopathy' or 'Machiavellianism' (terms associated with literature on the 'dark side') or simply to their bad character. But there is little evidence that bad people account for much of the conflict in the world, and a lot that all relationships can have a dark side. This is often defined as a combination of something that many psychologists, erroneously in my view, call psy.

Psychotherapists' work often brings them into contact with the dark side of people and relationships, that is with the minority of close relationships and their effects that are negative and have the potential to cause harm.

Meta-narrative

Vygotsky (1966) noted how often we accompany our actions with conversation, either with other people or, if we are on our own, with ourselves. We do not just talk to ourselves, in the 'inner speech' that Vygotsky described; we gesture too. Many people who are threading a needle, or driving a car through a narrow gap, find themselves putting their tongue out between their closed lips as if mimicking the action. Although we are much less likely to talk out loud or use extravagant gestures when we are alone, there is a continuity in these conversations from talking to others to talking to ourselves. We can carry on arguing with people even when the person is no longer physically there, and we can condemn ourselves too when we are on our own, just as we might do if we are being taken to task by someone else. We can also rehearse the viewpoints of what commonsense psychology calls the 'two minds' that we might be in.

The ambivalence of being in two minds can be a source of akrasia, but cannot explain the kind of akrasia that Camus attributed to seeing life as 'absurd', Marx and others attributed to alienation, or Sartre and many others attributed to meaninglessness. In Camus's (1960) masterpiece, *l'Etranger (The Outsider)*, the Algerian protagonist, Meursault, cannot look after his elderly mother, who goes into a home (he says they have nothing left to say to each other); visits occasionally; goes to her funeral but cannot understand why he should cry as all of us die; accepts a cup of coffee and smokes a cigarette during the vigil over her body but does not want to have the coffin lid taken off so that he can see her;

goes swimming with a girl (Marie) whose body he desires and makes love to her the day after the funeral; agrees with a neighbour who beats his dog that it is very sad when the dog runs off; is non-committal when his girlfriend asks him to marry her; agrees to write a letter to try to exculpate another neighbour who has beaten up the girl he prostitutes; goes to the beach with his girlfriend and drinks a lot; gets involved in a fight on behalf of a pimp; later feels the sun is beating him to his knees; sees one of the Arabs that he has been fighting produce a knife; realizes he could step back or step forward and shoot; steps forward and shoots but then pauses and empties his borrowed revolver into the man; finds people friendly to him in jail but cannot explain his motive for the killing and rejects absolution from the chaplain; is eventually found guilty of murder rather than an impulsive killing because of the extra shots; is portrayed by the prosecutor as what some people would currently call a 'psychopath' (Camus just uses the term 'heartless criminal'); and is then publicly beheaded by guillotine.

The white heat that engulfs Meursault is, I think, symbolic of a moment of crisis, in which choices have to be made. Meursault chooses to shoot but cannot ever say why. The court also has to choose and chooses to construct Meursault as a 'soulless monster' who sought out the Arab in order to kill him because of the earlier fight – although the main evidence for this is not any kind of expressed intention for revenge or any gain, but that Meursault had buried his mother in a heartless way. Evil does not really explain the murder since evil is not a motive. Camus (1960) wants us to take Meursault's point of view against the court, which is portrayed as unconcerned with Meursault at the end: the prosecutor even conflates Meursault's case with that of one due to be heard the following day.

Meursault's actions clearly belong on the dark side of human nature. Other people's indifference to him, including that of his mother, is an indication of the dark side of relationships, which I discuss below. Marie cares for him, but he is unable to see it, and she is unable to articulate it. Meursault's judgement about the other people in his life is flawed (it is not entirely clear if Marie does care for him or not). He attacks the chaplain who wants to offer him comfort, but believes the prosecutor who is building a devastating case against him; he categorizes his employer, who actually wants to help him and offers him a job in Paris, as exploitative. Yet, when facing death, Meursault realizes for the first time that he was sometimes happy in his former life, and he misses Marie's smile and her clothing.

Meursault is healthy, and in retrospect believes he was and is happy, once he had laid himself 'open for the first time to the benign indifference of the world. And finding it so much like myself, in fact so fraternal' (p. 120). The only thing he finally wanted was to overcome his loneliness by having a big crowd at his beheading, and for them to roar out with hate against him.

Overlaying the drama of Meursault's life is a meta-narrative that is never stated and which has to be created by the reader. This is a situation often confronted by the psychotherapist. A person may consult a psychotherapist about a lack of well-being, and present their life as a series of happenings, some of them unfortunate or having unhappy consequences, but these happenings are not apparently intended or deliberate. The task of the psychotherapist is, at least for many psychotherapists, to co-create with the client a narrative that provides a meta-narrative leading to greater well-being (Tantam, 2002).

Meursault is a personification of akrasia. He drifts through life going along with others simply because they ask it of him. His only positive action is to give in to aggression and murder someone, but he leaves it to others to deal with the consequences. Meursalt provides no narrative to account for his torpor. This kind of akrasia goes beyond the conscious struggles depicted in the dramaturgical model, to something deeper, and psychotherapists often find the clues for this in early life experience, nowadays often coupling this with the basic stuff – temperament and so on – that early life experience works on and with (Pressman et al., 2013), although this does not account for the reduced well-being created by infectious disease.

Early experience and well-being

Psychotherapy has focused especially on early life relationships because these are assumed to cast a shadow, or a light, over all subsequent relationships. This is probably due to two of Freud's key ideas: transference, which means that a pattern of relationships may persist throughout life with newly met people being pressed into the old pattern, rather than enabling a new one; and 'fixation'. Fixation was Freud's term for what happened when something stopped sexual development. Originally, the something was a precocious sexual awakening (Freud was very suspicious of chambermaids in this regard), although it might also be triggered by Freud's idea that sons were in love with their mothers until a fateful developmental phase when they realized that father was there first.

Empirical research is nowhere near specific enough to be able to test Freud's supposition about patterns. The difficulty is similar to that in testing nominative determinism. Finding an isomorphism between a pattern in childhood and a pattern in adulthood is highly probable as there are very many possible patterns of relationship at both ages, and any childhood pattern could be isomorphic with any adult pattern. It is much more difficult to show that the childhood pattern has been fundamental in some way, and that it has resulted in the formation of the isomorphic adult pattern, which is also fundamental.

However, using much simpler typologies of childhood relationships has enabled empirical research. Such typologies have included:

1. deprived vs. non-deprived
2. abusive (sexual or physical) vs. non-abusive
3. insecurely attached vs. securely attached
4. high vs. low parental control
5. high vs. low emotional involvement

Some of these overlap.

Deprivation

Deprivation may entail a lack of physical care, of nutrition, of health care, of cognitive stimulation or of emotional interaction. The latter two have been highlighted in children who were placed in orphanages in Romania, Russia and Moldova during the 1980s. Some of these children were subsequently adopted by Western European families and their progress was compared over time to those who were not adopted. One finding, which should not have been so surprising in retrospect, was that these very seriously emotionally and intellectually deprived children had abnormalities in their brains. Some of these abnormalities could be reversed after adoption, but not all. The brain is more like a muscle than was once thought. If it is not exercised, it atrophies, or rather the white matter connections (Sheridan et al., 2012) that allow the mature brain to function efficiently, do not develop without stimulation.

Abuse

Abusive relationships in childhood include children being the recipients of out-of-the-ordinary physical punishment or violence, witnessing violence, exposure to explicit sexual activity and being involved in explicit sexual activity with adults or older children. These are all associated with an increased risk of negative feelings in adulthood (Sugaya et al., 2012), and therefore with reduced well-being including poorer health, but there is also an association with feeling internally torn between conflicting feelings. One of the most overt expressions of this is an increased risk of harming oneself. Psychotherapy can reduce negative feelings in people with a history of being abused (Stevenson, 1999). There have been no longer-term studies of well-being as a result of psychotherapy, but one study has shown that people become less emotionally torn and therefore bring less conflicted emotion to life's challenges (Perry & Bond, 2012). There is good evidence (Crane, 2008) that psychotherapy reduces the demand for health care, suggesting that psychotherapy has more general effects on health.

Attachment

There is no doubt that being emotionally deprived has serious emotional consequences and, indeed, cognitive consequences. It is likely that one of these cognitive consequences is attention deficit disorder. The effects of deprivation are probably greater in people with particular hereditary sub-types (alleles) of the genes coding for receptors in the brain (Mileva-Seitz et al., 2013). Attachment theory refers to a more limited interaction between parenting and the mental health of offspring. It is based on ethological observations of the 'bonds' between mother animals and their children, and on the fact that anxiety runs in families. One possible explanation of the latter is heredity, but another is that there is a disturbance in the bond between mother and child.

Bonding is mediated by nonapeptide transmitters in the mid-brain. When a child is born, its suckling reflex produces letdown of the mother's milk and this triggers a surge of oxytocin, if the child has the right smell, that leads to mother and child 'bonding'. There are other pathways to bonding, but the effect is that mother and child monitor their distance from each other and if this becomes too great, or if danger threatens, both seek to restore proximity. Coming together reduces anxiety, probably by a direct effect on the amygdala. Attachment theory suggests that if this process goes wrong in some way, the child is 'insecure', because she or he cannot rely on the mother's protection. Insecurely attached children may be over-anxious or 'avoidant' (that is, cut off emotionally) or a mixture of the two. The exact role that oxytocin plays in this process is under active investigation (Carter, 2013). Given (intranasally) to adults, it increases memories of care by a mother figure if the adult is secure, but increases memories of neglect by the mother figure if the adult is insecure (Bartz et al., 2010).

Attachment theorists consider that security and the different types of insecurity are 'styles' of reacting that persist into adult life, and that they have an important impact on the trustfulness, intimacy and satisfactoriness of relationships. There is some evidence for this although the effect is weak (Madigan et al., 2013), unsurprisingly, given the many other relationships that can happen along the way to affect a person's trust or capacity for intimacy. Even a small influence persisting over so many years suggests that attachment has a powerful influence on a child. However, an alternative explanation is that the link between a mother's insecurity and that of her child – one of the main types of evidence for attachment theory – is mediated by a third variable, such as that both have genes for anxiety-proneness (Kagan & Snidman, 1999).

Few studies have been carried out of insecurely attached children following them into adulthood, but there have been more of adults who remember their early childhood experiences. One of the most recent showed that adults with a wide range of psychiatric disorders reported different kinds of childhood adversity, and that the more kinds of adversity there were, the more likely was an adult disorder (Green et al., 2010). However, these adversities were non-specific: every adversity increased the risk of any adult disorder, and none were of a kind that a psychotherapist would recognize as particularly traumatic or difficult, given any of the theoretical models considered above.

How does the dramaturgical model explain akrasia?

Our ability to carry through our intentions, according to the dramaturgical model, will depend on the part that we are given to play and this will not be under our control as the actor playing, or creating, that part. The recent upswing in the achievements of genetics and of neuroscience has focused a lot on these determinants of the human drama. Akrasia, for example, has been attributed to impairments in the frontal lobe, where it is supposed that higher cognitive functions associated with 'will' might lie.

Focusing on genetics or the wiring of the brain is like focusing on the script of a play alone. First, to do so omits the many versions that scripts go through – just as genetic factors are modified by experience through 'epigenetics' – but also misses out on what many would consider the most important experience of seeing a play – the interpretation of the script by the director, designer and actors. In psychology, the word script has most often been applied to our disposition to perform emotionally in certain ways, and we might say that this corresponds in our dramaturgical metaphor to the shape of the performance as laid down by the director. But, on the night, even this may be superseded by the chemistry of the actors, just as we may rise to an occasion, seemingly surpassing what others would see as our capacity, or we may unexpectedly fail or falter.

Our performance of our script may lack determination, be ambivalent or uncertain and all of these factors may lead to akrasia, just as much as any deficit in our hard-wired reward circuits. We may feel pulled in different directions by the people around us and end up doing nothing. We may also feel pulled in different directions by conflicting voices in our inner narrative. Sometimes people experience this concretely and, like Piers Plowman (Langland, 2011), their actions are preceded by a debate about the right course of action involving our conscience, the temptor's voice, and so on. Akrasia may result from an inability to resolve this debate, and this is probably the closest to the kind of spiritual sloth that afflicted St Anthony when he first became a hermit in the Egyptian desert. Akrasia may follow, too, if 'the elephant in the room' is being ignored: that is, if one of the most striking features of a current situation is being avoided. One of my colleagues once visited a woman with depression at home, as she was said to be suicidal. He was delayed, it was quite late on a Friday when he arrived and he found the family plunged into a kind of torpor, which seemed to emanate from his patient. After a while, her husband said, 'Well, I'd best be going' and he left the house. No one commented until my colleague asked where he had gone. One of the children said, 'Oh, he's gone to his other family. He always does that at weekends'.

As we have seen, psychoanalysts attribute failure to name the elephant to 'repression', a term that several French psychoanalysts interpreted to mean not being named, or signified, thus coming close to a narrative approach except that they saw this as a failure of the person and not a consequence of the 'play'. Existential analysts consider that an unwillingness to name the elephant might be a kind of self-deception, because naming the elephant makes it impossible not to address the threat or challenge that it presents.

Self-deception

Self-deception is a difficult concept. Like Sartre's critique of Freud's hypothesis of the censor that stands between the conscious and the unconscious and seems to know both, but remains veiled itself, self-deception seems to mean that we know something about ourselves and then choose to un-know it (Mele, 2000).

Someone like Meursault – who sides with his neighbour even when the neighbour beats up a girl, or sympathizes with another neighbour who constantly abuses his dog, and even wants to be taken as an ordinary friendly person after he has shot a near stranger for no very good reason – must surely live in self-deception.

Perhaps a better way of putting it would be that Meursault lives as if he is not an agent who has an effect on other people. It is this that leads the prosecutor to think that he does not have a soul, and in a way the prosecutor is right, if we mean by soul the origin of accountable action.

There might be many reasons for repudiating agency. We might say that, like many of the defendants at the Nuremberg trials, we were simply following orders or fitting in with other people's expectations. Or we might say that we did not know what we were doing or did not see the implications or the effects. Perhaps it is possible to feel well-being even in the absence of agency, but it would be hard to claim satisfaction with life.

Irrationality

Like most other psychotherapists, I do not believe that emotions or 'irrationality' are our undoing. As the example of Meursault indicates, a lack of emotions – or at least a lack of awareness of our own emotions – may endanger our life satisfaction.

But there is no doubt that psychotherapists are familiar with people who cleave to a life of pain, anxiety or conflict, even if well-being is possible. Psychologists may think that this is mere ignorance and can be dealt with by education. Psychotherapists are much more willing to consider that people may not only be drawn to act in ways that decrease well-being, but will actively resist changing these actions even if others point out alternatives. Freud was so puzzled by what he called this 'repetition compulsion' that he took over the concept of his trainee (and Jung's patient, colleague and lover) Sabina Spielrein, that we are motivated by a 'death instinct' as well as a love instinct.

I find proponents of thinking positively through determined self-improvement ingenuous because they do not recognize this dark side of irrationality, assuming that once people are told what to do, they will just do it. Generally, clients who engage with positive therapists are willing to obey the authority of the therapists and improve themselves. Perhaps those whose natures are more complex and conflicted are less likely to consult a positive psychologist, and so the positive psychologist does not need a theory to take the tragic side of human nature into account.

Never being able to forgive

One reason that people live with grief, disappointment or hate is that they feel that they have to live up to the claim, 'I will never forgive him/her for what he/she did' (Seawell et al., 2013). Forgiveness is beneficial to the forgiver – it improves cardiovascular health, for example (Larsen et al., 2012) – but it seems to allow the offending person to go unpunished. Being unforgiving is a bit like seeking revenge: it is driven by a sense of justice that is more important than mere well-being. The pursuit of vengeance may destroy a person's life and put the person's family at risk if a round of retaliation is started up.

One reason for pursuing a self-destructive course knowingly may be to maintain a victim status that says to the world, 'Look how I have been left'. Being unforgiving may bring destruction. A patient of mine was walking to work, very early in the morning, when a lorry mounted the pavement and he was hit. The crush fracture of his leg failed to heal and he had to have an amputation. He refused to get a prosthesis fitted, arguing that he wanted to see justice done before he got on with his life. A protracted legal action followed, with a settlement in his favour but much smaller, and much later, than he thought he deserved. Tragically, he developed an osteosarcoma in the stump before he could get a prosthesis and he died of the tumour.

Like the man who wears a placard saying, 'wife and children to support' or the man we recently observed in Sheffield whose placard said 'I am not a drug user, but I am homeless and need money', the poor man who had so unfairly been knocked down was enacting a life story that he thought must be told, but he did this at the expense of a happier story of his life.

Gustavo Berti and his wife Alicia Schneider-Berti created Renacer, following the death of their 18-year-old son. Renacer has now grown to 120 self-help groups for bereaved parents. The couple write (personal communication, 2011): 'All bereaved parents ask what meaning is left in life. Some fear the existential vacuum perceived just ahead, while others realize for the first time that it has always been their road companion'.

I will consider the meaning vacuum in the next chapter, but here I want to quote from Gustavo and Alicia's experience in another way. They note that many parents bereaved in this way feel that grieving is a way of demonstrating the severity of their loss, and that stopping grieving makes light not only of their own feelings but of their dead child's value – as if it implies that the child did not matter enough for the grieving to be endless. But sooner or later, with the encouragement of others in the Renacer groups, some parents can see that they are thereby 'allowing our life to be destroyed by the very person we love the most' (personal communication, 2011): that their child would not want his or her parents to waste the remainder of their lives in grief.

Vengeance, grief, nostalgia and regret are examples of emotions that involve hoping that some future action can put the past 'right'. The two examples we have considered show clearly that the past cannot be changed, but only how we remember it. So making the past right does not work, only making ourselves right with the past. Self-deception in all its various forms is a way of trying to change the present without changing ourselves in relation to the facts of the present.

9

No Viewpoint

Life satisfaction is yet another measure of the combination of happiness, health and morality (I have presented so many such combinations to the reader that I felt the need to summarize them, in Box 9.1). Life satisfaction takes account not just of how people feel about their life, but also of what they think about it. Two influential researchers in happiness, Seligman and Diener, have each moved away from an exclusive focus on positive feelings and well-being to life satisfaction as a better measure of what they would consider 'the good life'. Seligman currently defines this as requiring five dimensions of living: positive emotion; engagement; relationships; meaning; and achievement involving the application of determination (Seligman, 2011).

Albert Einstein (1930) believed in determination too, but his values otherwise seem very different (Einstein, 1930). What made his life satisfying was not his achievement, which he described as '[a] few ideas to which I have with my feeble powers attained through ceaseless struggle' (1930: 193), but his value to others, particularly to the community of scholars to which he belonged. And he excoriated people who 'looked upon ease and happiness as ends in themselves – such an ethical basis I call the ideal of a pigsty' (p. 193).

BOX 9.1

Happiness 1 (Hedonic): Awareness of pleasurable feelings
Happiness 2 (Eudaimonic, subjective well-being): Disposition to experience pleasurable feelings
Well-being: Happiness and health combined
Quality of life: Happiness, health and the absence of pain or disability
Life satisfaction: Positive appraisal of conduct in and circumstances of life, usually but not always associated with a good quality of life.

Life satisfaction takes account of how well a person judges they have accomplished the goals in life that they have chosen, or accepted, as being the most valuable. The ability to control one's life is an important determinant of how well people can deliberately achieve a goal and so is linked to life satisfaction (Wiest et al., 2013). Goals are often material (Luhmann et al., 2012) and so life satisfaction is increased by material wealth (Diener et al., 2010) in a way that well-being is not. Life satisfaction is strongly correlated with social class and income. As the economists note, worldly success is only satisfying if one has kept up with the Joneses. Life satisfaction has tended therefore to remain stable in European countries like Finland (Koivumaa-Honkanen et al., 2005), even though more and more powerful goods have been accumulated by most households. In Finland, this has meant that a minority of the population have remain locked in a life situation that they consider unsatisfactory, however.

Life satisfaction has been used in national surveys, for example in the UK by the Department for Environment, Food and Rural Affairs (http://sd.defra.gov.uk/2010/07/wellbeing-statistics/) and by the UN Office for Economic Cooperation and Development (www.oecdbetterlifeindex.org/topics/life-satisfaction/), who publish a league table of life satisfaction, country by country.

The life satisfaction scale developed by Diener et al. (1985), succeeding their subjective well-being scale, has been widely used in psychology research, most usually as a means of estimating the average life satisfaction in populations. It has been used less often as a means of finding out what makes an individual's life satisfying, although there have been studies showing an association with gratitude (Wood et al., 2008) and appreciation (Fagley, 2012). Interestingly, these associations apply even if appreciation is only evinced in day-dreams (Mar et al., 2012). I suppose this is because we are only too willing to tell ourselves how grateful or appreciative someone would be of our efforts 'if they only knew' how much we have done for them.

The associations with appreciation and gratitude indicate that other people's appraisals of our value are linked to our own appraisals of ourselves but, for many philosophers, this has not been enough. The saying of Socrates that 'the unexamined life is not worth living' was repeated by Kierkegaard, among others, to indicate that he believed that life satisfaction based on our standing in the social world was, in some way, inferior to life satisfaction based on our own valuation of ourselves. We should, he thought, weigh ourselves up independently and come to our own conclusions about how satisfied we should be with our lives.

Seligman, whose work I have often had occasion to quote in the last few chapters, considered that the unexamined life was a life stuck at the stage of the pleasant life (Seligman, 2003). He postulated two further stages: the good life and the meaningful life. These are the same stages that Kierkegaard had proposed some 150 years before. Kierkegaard called them the aesthetic, the ethical and the religious stages on life's way (Kierkegaard, 1988 (1844)). The religious stage, Kierkegaard thought, could not be reached by following conventional ethical formulae, but by a 'leap of faith'. For Kierkegaard, it required the discovery of a personal faith in God, and not just cleaving to the established church.

The aesthetic life and the ethical life stages both meant living according to other people's rules or values: good taste in the former, conventional ethics in the latter. Leading life according to these precepts does not require the deepest kind of examination that Kierkegaard ultimately gave to his own life, and that of the religious luminaries around him.

The ethical life

The division between the aesthetic life and the ethical life is very similar to that between hedonic and eudaemonic happiness. I have presented many of the arguments in favour of the ethical life providing more lasting happiness than the aesthetic life in several chapters already. Aristotle was in favour of it providing more life satisfaction, too, since there was satisfaction to be gained from honing our innate abilities to a high level of skill, and life satisfaction in honing our capacity for living to its greatest expression.

Practising a skill is often traditionally defined. In Aristotle's day, the martial arts to which he sometimes refers as exemplars would certainly have been so governed. If one is born into a culture with traditions about living of this kind, life satisfaction can be most easily achieved, I would suppose, if one follows Aristotle's precepts.

Kierkegaard concluded that the ethical life was not good enough for him, and he took his contemporaries to task for being satisfied with living comfortably as well as ethically. One of his targets, Grundtvig (Allchin, 1997), has, like Kierkegaard, gained enduring fame. Like Kierkegaard, he had a spiritual crisis but seems to have emerged from it without deviating from his course of life. Grundtvig's life gradually became less turbulent as he got older, a not unusual happening in people who become more satisfied in their older years (Westermeyer, 2013). His views became more liberal, he embraced the Lutheran establishment and it, in turn, embraced him.

Older people with high life satisfaction are more likely to have maintained an active sex life (Woloski-Wruble et al., 2010) and Grundtvig was no exception. He married for the third time at the age of 76. Older people who are satisfied with their lives continue to be active in other ways (Ni Mhaolain et al., 2012), exercising their minds as well as their brains (Enkvist et al., 2013). Grundtvig adhered to this pattern. He gave his last sermon a few days before his death at the age of 89. Unlike Kierkegaard, he followed in the path that his father wanted for him, and his son took up Grundtvig's interest in folklore and, unlike Kierkegaard, but like other older satisfied people (H.-C. Hsu, 2010), he is unlikely to have wanted for material comfort.

Gods, or God, and the ethical life

Religions provide the traditions that direct many of us on how to lead an ethical life and thereby achieve life satisfaction. For those who acknowledge them, they are powerfully backed by a divinity with the power to see ends to life that are obscure to their followers. The divinity communicates this knowledge through a third party, sometimes nameless or sometimes identified as an angel or, in the case of the 12 commandments, a burning bush. Whatever or whoever, the intermediary claims this same knowledge of where actions will take us in this life, or, in some religions, in later lives. To be a useful guide to life, divine sayings must be interpreted and turned into detailed prescriptions for living by faith communities. It is not easy to put these prescriptions into practice and they chafe. Grundtvig, for example, fell foul of his church and had to go home to a living provided by his father in the early part of his career. People who do not lose faith in a tradition, and accept and abide by its ethical directives, are more likely to be able to draw on it in later life to achieve greater life satisfaction, even though they may recognize that it is insufficient (Fletcher, 2004) and that they may have to alter their memories to make them compatible with key points of doctrine (Seligman, 2005).

How to gain life satisfaction after losing faith

For the many millions who more or less follow this traditional path, there are many other millions for whom the thread of traditional belief is broken. This may happen to believers as well as non-believers if believers reject the interpretation of God's will provided by their faith community.

Kierkegaard was one of these. He thought that a true religious life could only begin when a person found God for themselves. Kierkegaard was trained to be a minister in the established church of his time and could have stayed in it, as his brother did. Whether he chose not to, or whether he could not fit into it because of his unwillingness to go along with any group, is hard to say. For whatever reason, he became a path-breaker. Not everyone can choose to break a new path, as Kierkegaard did. Many people experience a break in their expected life course as a result of a loss of faith, or of a disaster, passion or rejection. What they have in common with Kierkegaard is that they can no longer rely on the life satisfaction that comes from aiming and achieving the goals that they have previously shared with their traditional community.

Kierkegaard imagined this kind of break as both a leap and a fall. This is how Kierkegaard described the life of the person who is truly worthy (in his opinion), the Knight of Infinity or, as he more often called the role, the Knight of Faith (Kierkegaard, 1843/1983):

> Most people live dejectedly in worldly sorrow and joy; they are the ones who sit along the wall and do not join in the dance. The knights of infinity are dancers and possess elevation. They make the movements upward and fall down again. But whenever they fall down they are not able at once to assume the posture, they vacillate an instant, and this vacillation shows that after all they are strangers in the world (ibid., p. 29).

Kierkegaard may have been thinking of some of history's great prophets when writing this. Those people who make a leap of faith often do so in order to recover from a fall, a fall that may indicate an unlucky disaster but also a limitation in their personality: their 'coping ability', as we should say. Gautama Buddha walked out on his family and on being next in line to the throne of his North Indian principality. Jesus Christ was unpopular in his home town of Nazareth and wandered into the desert. The Prophet Mohammed began to hear the voice of the angel Gabriel that drove him to sermonize against his fellow citizens who repeatedly tried to kill him as a result.

Falling is the inevitable concomitant of leaping. As the French say about depression, 'on doit reculer pour mieux sauter': 'it's necessary to draw back to jump further'. Depression and Kierkegaard's 'falling' have many resemblances (Gall, 2006), except that one falls with the intention of rising again.

Falls can be destructive but they can also be transformative – so long, that is, if one can find a new path towards life satisfaction. Finding a new path after a crisis that has vitiated former life goals or has blocked any possible path to them is therefore a priority. The question is, how can one do that?

Turning to God

Turning to God or simply turning inward (Stonington, 2011) is a common way to find a new path. One study cites a figure of 39% of people diagnosed with HIV who report a spiritual transformation (Ironson & Kremer, 2009). Nearly half of people who consult traditional healers report persistent spiritual change, and improvements in their health have been attributed to this (Mainguy et al., 2013).

Some people are able to find positive meaning even in dying of cancer (Ando et al., 2012), but other people feel that this and other catastrophes that break the thread of an accustomed life, leach away the meaning that life has had. Many people in this situation have turned for inspiration to a book by an Austrian Jewish psychiatrist who lost his wife, parents and other members of his family in the Holocaust and who himself survived the concentration camps. Victor Frankl (1963) had to deal with losing the meaning of his life as a result of his experiences, but had probably done so before, as an adolescent, when he contemplated the point of life. Some years after this, he created a student counselling service for other suicidal students, and it seems that one of the most enduring things in his life that gave him meaning was being a healer – a link with Bentham and his view that increasing the happiness of others increases one's own.

Frankl's (1963) book about his experiences was called, in English, *Man's Search for Meaning*, and in his many lectures and television experiences he stressed that well-being required one to have a meaningful life. He founded a school of psychotherapy, logotherapy, which specializes in helping people to discover a stronger sense of meaning.

So, what is the meaning of life?

The problem with this approach is that it relies on both therapist and client knowing what kind of a thing the meaning of life is. Charles Dickens, whose avowed views about the meaning of Christmas have influenced many English-speaking families, put into David

Copperfield's mouth the idea that the meaning of life was to put in effort: Copperfield says, in Chapter 42 of the eponymous book:

> My meaning simply is, that whatever I have tried to do in life, I have tried with all my heart to do well; that whatever I have devoted myself to, I have devoted myself to completely; that in great aims and in small, I have always been thoroughly in earnest.

Dickens is often quoted as finding life a grind, although these are actually words put in the mouth of Mr Mantalini in Nicholas Nickleby. Some humanistic psychologists have assumed, though, that authors use their characters to express their own beliefs and analysed the content of 238 quotations, including quotations of characters as well as the authors themselves (Kinnier et al., 2003). The quotations were contributed by 195 'eminent people' and Dickens was placed in the group voicing the sixth commonest theme extracted: that life is a struggle. The ten themes that the authors extracted were:

1. To enjoy or experience life (the most common and found in 17% of quotes);
2. To love, help, or serve others. This group included quotes from Gandhi, J. Rousseau and Einstein;
3. Life is a mystery. Camus, Kierkegaard, and, again, Einstein contributed quotes to this group;
4. Life is meaningless. 11% of the quotes had this content and, as one might expect, Schopenhauer, Kafka and Sartre quotes were also attributed to this theme, but so were quotes by Freud and the noted humourist, H. L. Mencken;
5. To serve or worship God and/or prepare for the next (or after-) life. Quotes from Gandhi, well known spiritual leaders and less expectedly Nelson Mandela and Thomas Paine were placed here;
6. Life is a struggle. As well as the Nickleby quote, there were quotes here, too, from Benjamin Disraeli, George Bernard Shaw, and Jonathan Swift;
7. To contribute to something that is greater than ourselves. Quotes here from Emerson and Benjamin Franklin, but also William Faulkner, Margaret Mead, Richard Nixon, and the popular writer on philosophy, Will Durant;
8. To become self-actualized. Included here are quotes from Thoreau, Plato, Nietzsche, and Marie Curie as well as the novelist Robert Louis Stevenson;
9. To create your own meaning. Quotes by Simone de Beauvoir, Viktor Frankl, and Carl Jung figure here; the final group included quotes on the theme that
10. Life is absurd or a joke. Quotes were contributed here from a comedian, Charlie Chaplin, a wit, Oscar Wilde, and a philosopher, Camus.

Both of these ideas about meaning, getting an A for effort or an A for achievement, presuppose that one is somehow engaged with life and moving towards some identifiable end. But this sense of a goal disappears when life becomes really meaningless. Both Camus (1960), who described life as absurd, and Sartre (1969), who wrote 'it is meaningless that we are born; it is meaningless that we die' (ibid., p. 547), thought that even the scraps of meaning that Dickens allowed were arbitrary. Whilst we agree with Sartre's reasoning, it seems to vitiate much of what we have said so far about living well. It runs counter to Frankl's (1963) idea that we cannot live without meaning; it strikes against the prudential nature of eudaimonia; and it seems to make a nonsense of our efforts to improve our health. Both Sartre and Camus won Nobel prizes for literature. Both were active, politically engaged figures. So their view that life is meaningless or absurd seems to run counter to the highly engaged way in which they themselves lived. What could they have meant?

Where is my life going?

Sartre (1969) recognized that it is not possible to live satisfactorily without having goals, but he also thought that we should be ready to dispense with them. Recent research supports this and also supports Sartre's idea that living according to social prohibitions is not conducive to flourishing (Elliot et al., 2012). Camus sometimes referred to his formative experience as a goalkeeper in a successful university football team, where goals were the be all and end all. Camus's football career was ended by TB, so he was well aware that nothing was destined, nothing good could be taken for granted. Sartre (ibid.) believed that nothing in our lives was fore-ordained: any goal that we aimed for could turn out very differently to our expectations. It was for this reason that he thought that our being was 'nothing' until we created it through our actions. How we end up at the end of lives, what kind of being we are, will be a product of these actions or choices, but it is not like a sculpture that we can create. In fact, it is more like what undertaking a commission does to the sculptor. We might aim to be a good parent and end up being known by our children as a disciplinarian – or we may discover, looking back, that we were a good parent. The best that we can do is to project ourselves into the future and ask, 'if I continue like this, what will my life have looked like?' Hence my title for this chapter: in Sartre's world, our viewpoint is always looking back – there is no viewpoint on the future at all.

A common response to Sartre was to accuse him of tearing up ethics. 'Anything goes' was the slogan that seemed to apply. Religious commentators pointed out that our god or gods had set out the proper aims and conduct of life, and that one indispensable goal of living was to obey them. Other people were concerned that Sartre, in his remorseless concentration (particularly in the *Critique of Dialectical Reason*) (Sartre, 2004) on power and its inescapability was endorsing a dog-eat-dog world view that took no account of the finer feelings, like altruism. Sartre was scathing about altruism and religion (although not about the pseudo-religion of Marxism). Actually, Sartre's ethics were even more remorseless than those of many religions. There were no prizes for good intentions. We are judged on who we have been, whatever we wanted or tried to be. Sartre judged himself rather leniently, but history has judged him more harshly and many have concluded that he lived an immoral life.

Are man or woman divine that they can see the ends of their actions?

Why should I be concerning myself with this now neglected, and arguably immoral, novelist, philosopher and political activist? One reason is that the neglect of his philosophical work does not reflect its value, which is in need of re-estimation. But the main one is that his belief that life is meaningless, coupled with his disgust at his physical self, are characteristics of a particular kind of ill being that is different from any that we have considered in previous chapters, but is common nonetheless. It is the kind of ill being that leads a young person to harm her- or himself, for example by cutting into their wrists or upper thigh, or an older person to drink too much, night after night. It cannot be attributed to poor health or even to unhappiness or a lack of satisfaction with achievement. It is more profound than this, affecting all of what Emmy van Deurzen (2009) calls the four worlds of being: physical, social, psychological and spiritual. If there were parallel universes, and an individual could move between them (which would of course obviate the point of postulating parallel universes), it might be the feeling we would have if we were moved from our present universe and dropped into a different one. It is the feeling that we do not belong, do not fit in, have the wrong smell, that everything smells wrong around us, that we are not fully present, that we are different in an obviously alien way, that we are a different race.

Many modernist writers have expressed these feelings in different ways. They are apparent in Tolstoy's later work, notably *The Death of Ivan Ilyitch*. Robert Musil's *Man without Qualities* experiences them, as does Kafka's insect who has metamorphosed from a man. The philosopher Kierkegaard had them, and with his brother put them down to a curse laid on his father and his father's children.

We could, as some commentators do, put these feelings down to a kind of intellectual sickness. Healthy people, such commentators say, know where they are going, know that it is right to be going there and put their backs into the effort to reach their goal as soon as possible. We are not convinced by these arguments. We are only too aware that people who have visions of the future can easily be deceived by them. One definition of a god is that they and they alone can foresee the consequences of human action. For the rest of us, we have to accept that actions may have quite unforeseen consequences. Goals are a bit like the preface to a book: one writes the preface as if it precedes the book but, in fact, it is usually written after the book is completed. This becomes most obvious when the goals that we adopt turn out to be unattainable.

Values and the death of the soul

Sartre challenges our accustomed ideas about life-span development in another way. Not only does he challenge the idea that we can, without being in bad faith, have goals, but he also challenges the idea that we are in the driving seat of our development. In fact, he suggests that no one is driving. If this were taken to its extreme, then there would be no Jean-Paul Sartre or Digby Tantam at all – just an empty body being bumped and bashed through life, like a bumper car at a circus.

Clearly, Sartre cannot mean this. So we need to ask ourselves what it is that holds a life together. Sartre was fascinated by this and wrote several 'psychobiographies', including his own (*Les Mots*) (Sartre, 1964) for which he won a Nobel Prize for Literature.

Sartre was influenced by Heidegger, although Heidegger himself rejected Sartre's existentialism. Heidegger goes as far as he can in *Being and Time* to strip away some of our preconceptions about existence (the everyday meaning of Dasein) in order to bring out its fundamental nature. He gives considerable space to the problem of time. Suppose I had Korsakoff psychosis, which meant I could remember new facts only so long as I kept thinking of them. Someone with Korsakoff psychosis cannot remember what they had for lunch, for example, unless they write it down. How could I know I was Digby? Heidegger splits this problem into an ontic one and, what he calls, an ontological one. Ontically, I might note that people called me Digby, that I had belongings which had the Digby name on them or that my driver's license said I was Digby. But if that were all, my experience of being Digby would be no different from the experience of being Digby yesterday, John today and Jim tomorrow. So what goes beyond this ontic experience that makes me think that whatever I am called or whatever I am wearing, I am fundamentally me and will remain me? This, for Heidegger, is an ontological question, about the fundamentals of existence.

Our usual conception of ourselves is here and now: how we feel, what we plan, who we think fondly of, how our body feels, and so on NOW. We can remember some of these sensations, emotions and thoughts from yesterday but we do not experience them.

But the question arises, why are we Fred or Maria or Wilhelm today and also tomorrow? Fred today may be hungry, disappointed and hopeless. Fred tomorrow may be well fed, satisfied and cheerful. How can we know that Fred today is the same person as Fred tomorrow? One answer is that we have the same identity and that we would therefore pass identity checks. But if we found that we had forgotten all our correct PIN codes, our keys did not open our own front door, our children or friends did not recognize us, would we calmly say, obviously we are not the same person? We don't normally prove our identity on a regular basis, to check that it hasn't changed. We normally think of ourselves as continuously existing. As Heidegger writes, we normally think of ourselves as projected in time, as four-dimensional in fact.

So what aspect of our being projects in time? Clearly, it is not simply our appearance because if we were to superimpose pictures of ourselves from every birthday, we would see at best a family resemblance and if we had the misfortune to have had major surgery on our face, not necessarily even that. Some of our relationships may remain constant over many years, but this may not be true of everyone. Our DNA remains the same, or so we assume, but it may be expressed differently at different ages. Anyway, we are not aware of our DNA profile and we may not be aware of having a particular temperament either. So we cannot rely on them as cues for us to know that we are the same person. People do not think very often about whether they wake up the same person as they went to bed. However, when the direction of life has taken a new turn, these are the questions that people ask.

I think that what makes people feel they remain the same person is that they experience the world as being unchanged. Our convictions about the world still hold, and we cherish some of them with more emotional intensity than others such that some of them are constitutive of what we really believe or who we really are. But, even these values may change and we may then rightly say, 'I am not the same person. I've changed. I'm not the person I was'.

In 1981, Illinois Bell Telephone sacked almost half of its workforce of 26,000. At the time, Salvatore Maddi, a social psychologist, had been working with about 450 executives for the previous six years, and many of them were in the group that were sacked. Maddi and his co-workers followed the sacked executives for up to a further six years (Maddi & Kobasa, 1984). According to Maddi, about two thirds of them developed health problems and a third apparently thrived. There was no control group, so it is not clear what proportion of people of their age would have developed health problems anyway, but Maddi concluded that there was an excess of problems due to the upheaval, in combination with what he and his co-workers called a lack of 'hardiness'. Hardy people were committed to projects; considered stress to be a challenge to overcome; and had a belief that they could control even the effects of bad things happening. These beliefs were unchanged by the upheaval, but the beliefs of the other two thirds were uprooted.

Losing meaning, goals or values clearly destroys the life satisfaction of many, and, if Maddi's conclusions are correct, may even be fatal. There is a parallel with experiments on dogs conducted by Seligman and Maier (Seligman, 1967) in which dogs that were given intermittent electric shocks that were turned off by another dog, but could not be turned off by themselves, developed 'learned helplessness', demonstrated in a later experiment by showing that these dogs did not jump off an electrified plate, even though they could, but just laid down and whined. As in the Maddi experiment, about a third of dogs that had the uncontrolled shocks did not become helpless, however, and Seligman concluded that these dogs were optimistic.

A very different explanation for both experiments is that belief in oneself, coupled with depreciatory beliefs about others, are not going to be challenged by being sacked – they may even be reinforced. So 'hardiness' may be spurious: it may just be that, for these people, this particular situation did not destroy their beliefs. Those people whose beliefs were destroyed may have been better employees, since they apparently believed less in personal control or fighting against adversity. Dogs do not have beliefs – or do they? Some dogs believe that people will care for them and repay that with acceptance. These are, on the whole, good dogs to have. A dog like that, though, might be defeated by suddenly discovering that they are trapped in a laboratory where they are regularly given electric shocks without having done anything to justify being punished.

I believe that Maddi and Seligman were, in different ways, denying the importance of good or bad fortune by arguing that the intrinsic capacities of their executives or their dogs could determine an outcome. But their studies did demonstrate that when people, or dogs, are deprived of control over events, they are particularly vulnerable, and this has been borne out by other research on redundancy (Price et al., 2002). Taking away a person's control means that they are no longer able to strive for their goals, or to impose their own values, and for many of us who, like Sartre, take free choice to be the pre-requisite of giving meaning to life, losing our autonomy also challenges life's meaning.

Vulnerability

I differ from the positive psychologists who seem to assume that we are always in control of our own being. I differ from the doctors who think that when we are not in control, it is always because we have developed a kind of illness (although that *may* be the case). I recognize that a temporary loss of well-being may become an enduring one, and that this happens to many people who are defeated by life. I would dearly love to say that one might inject this or that meaning back into a person's life or give them some new goal, or that the values of this religion or that great writer will revitalize them, but I do not believe this to be true.

So what can a carer, a therapist or a professional do when faced with someone in this state? Clearly, people in this state are vulnerable. Indeed, some may be so terrified that they actually think they are dying. Having lost their identity, people in this kind of existential crisis are easy prey to people with answers or solutions. Clearly, too, there is a potential for transformation in the longer term. I think that all that can, and should, be offered is care, but that care needs to be of a personal and not technical nature. It takes someone who has themselves been through the terror of transformation to hold someone who is still going through it.

Passion

Despite the terror of transformation, despite the risks to well-being, people still seek out existential crises, even when the crises do not come to them. Sometimes this works out well. Psychologists and psychiatrists often use group averages in their research, and this has led to a focus on a kind of normalized trajectory of human life. So when positive psychologists recommend what is best for well-being, they are often assuming that they are addressing someone with the expectation that they will progress through life with an average trajectory. Psychotherapists, however, are much more used to dealing with people who have veered off the average trajectory, and it is often a passion that has caused them to do so.

Living a life without passion sometimes seems worse than putting everything in one's life in jeopardy. T.S. Eliot captures this living deadness in his poem, *The Hollow Men* (Eliot, 1969), which he wrote when his marriage was breaking up, his estranged first wife was developing a psychiatric disorder and he had failed to complete his first verse drama, *Sweeney Agonistes* (ibid.). A year after its publication, he joined the Anglican communion and remained a devoted Anglo-Catholic thereafter.

The Hollow Men begins:

We are the hollow men

We are the stuffed men

Leaning together

Headpiece filled with straw.

Alas!

> Our dried voices, when
>
> We whisper together
>
> Are quiet and meaningless
>
> As wind in dry grass
>
> Or rats' feet over broken glass
>
> In our dry cellar. (ibid., p. 87)

However, we rarely need to seek passion out: it finds us. Passions are strong emotions that act as motivators. They are by no means always lustful. The notion that great ambition is the passion of great character is often attributed to Napoleon but there is no evidence that he actually said it. Henry James definitely wrote that doubt was, although he put the sentiment in the mouth of a fictional writer, Dencombe. Albert Camus wrote that passion was a taste for truth (1960), and Kierkegaard that it was faith (Kierkegaard, 1843/1983). Rage is a passion, and so is revenge, as Samuel Johnson pointed out (Johnson, 1839). Passion often involves suffering (Eliot compared it to a toothache) (Eliot, 1989). Many writers who have discussed passion agree with Napoleon Bonaparte who thought that passion either made people do very good or very bad acts. One of the very bad acts that passion is often credited with is to be half-hearted. Passions may cause people to smash their present world, but may not give them enough energy to build a new one. Aristotle thought that passions (pathoi) clouded reason but that well-developed reason would always see through the actions that passions dictated unless a person was too impetuous, too improvident, to think or was so weak (or akratic – we discussed this in the last chapter) that they could not back up the recommendations of their own reason. Either way, passion was dangerous and best avoided – as we noted Socrates advising Heracles in Chapter 1.

This distrust of passion has been shared by many philosophers since Socrates and Aristotle, perhaps not surprisingly since they were in the business of selling Reason. Master Kong, Gautama Buddha and the anonymous transmitters of the Vedas agreed with Western philosophy in this, considering that practising exactly the kind of continence that Aristotle and Socrates valued would lead to goodness and freedom from reincarnation, whilst also recognizing that passion was needed for creation and was important to the family man who could not pursue continence to the same degree as the holy man who withdraws from life.

'Staying cool'

One way of dealing with passion is to avoid emotion even if this means, as it often does, avoiding engagement. Although only a minority of people might endorse avoiding all emotions, many people might be encouraged by positive psychologists to do such a thing. Staying cool is often interpreted to mean staying fixed in one part of what I call the 'emotional compass'.

E-motions are movements, as the name indicates, but this movement has been difficult to capture within the psychology tradition of quantitative research, where a daily average of emotion has proved most useful in well-being research, as we discussed in Chapter 3. Snapshots and averages do not capture the mobility, flexibility and creativity of emotional life, any more than a still of a ballet can do any more than hint at the whole performance. Research on emotional expressions demonstrates that dynamic portrayals of emotions, for example in videos, produce more activation than still photographs (Recio et al., 2011) and therefore lead to more accurate processing (Trautmann et al., 2009) that is more closely integrated with socially important information, such as gaze direction (Sato et al., 2010).

Watching, or experiencing, a dynamic display such as dance activates the right parietal cortex (Grosbras et al., 2012), an area of the brain where an increase in activation relative to the left cortex is associated with depression (Hecht, 2010). Activation of this area in the short term may lead to its longer-term inactivation, and this may be one means by which creative activities involving movement increase well-being. This would be close to Aristotle's idea that drama results in an emotional purge or κάθαρσις (catharsis).

Although there is good evidence, which I reviewed in Chapter 4, that anxiety reduces well-being, there is also evidence, as we noted previously, that a background level of anxiety is both normal and desirable. Terror management theory, like existential psychotherapy, attributes this to the fear of death. Terror management theory studies have also demonstrated that this anxiety does not grow and dominate awareness in normal circumstances, but is canalized into shoring up defences against an awareness of mortality. These defences are not necessarily at the expense of well-being and may sometimes enhance functioning that is known to increase well-being. For example, making someone more aware of their mortality may lead to enhanced well-being, closer relationships and more altruism (for reference to these and other effects, see Exhibit 31 in Bellen, 2010).

Emotions are, as I have already noted, in motion. A symphony, a popular song, a poem, all of these move forward, sometimes telling a story and sometimes not, but always having a characteristic emotional development. We give a great deal of attention to the formal structure of an argument, rather less to that of a chat and very little to this kind of emotional flow. However it, too, has a structure that Charles Sanders Peirce noted in his *Semiology* (Peirce, 1958). This was taken up by Freud who saw the two principles of Peirce's iconic and indexical signification – resemblance and synechdoche respectively – in the development of a dream and of symptoms during the natural history of a psychiatric disorder (Freud, 1913). Freud was the first, and possibly the most prolific, psychotherapist to trace emotional narratives in everyday life, from the dreams and symptoms of anxiety disorder already mentioned, to jokes, culture, literary texts and religions. Jung (1989) also made an important contribution to this field. Despite the ingenuity with which these links have been established, they have received little attention outside of psychotherapy. Perhaps one reason is that the plans that we hold in our attention can only span a short period, but emotional links may extend over much longer periods of time, as illustrated in the stream of consciousness novelistic device, for example in Virginia Woolf's novels.

I have argued that the flow of emotions is important in well-being and perhaps as important as their average value. This flow will encompass negative as well as positive emotions and this leads to a substantial difference in the approach to well-being of positive psychologists, who focus on emotional regulation designed to maintain a constant positive level of emotionality (Koole, 2008) and psychotherapists who aim at making emotions fluid, rather than being fixed in a negative (or a positive) direction.

Liberating passion and iron will

Passion, like other emotions, is a movement. Its dynamic effect may burst its bounds, break things up, clear blockages and move things along. It may scupper our best laid plans and our best attempts to create a persona that will impress or attract other people. The effects may be either negative or positive in the long run.

Theologians have been more confident about passion so long as the passion comes from a union with God, who guides and shapes it. Kierkegaard, boiling over with emotion as he was, was a passionate philosopher in this sense, as was Nietzsche who remained theological in his outlook, even though he had dispensed with God. Nietzsche put a hypostatized sense of destiny in place of God, usually translated into English as 'Will'. Will is closely related to Aristotelian continence and Nietzsche agreed with Aristotle that will could be strong or weak, just as passions are. The Ubermensch had strong passions which drove him (no mention of her) forward with energy and determinism, but they were directed by an even stronger will.

Nietzsche may have defined will as 'will to power' but his own life could be better described as will to utter the truth, like Camus (1960). Nietzsche did not, like Kierkegaard, have a spiritual authority or a central value – love in Kierkegaard's case – to fall back on. His own instincts were to submit, not to dominate. But the Nazis and other German militarists who cited his work but whose passion was to dominate demonstrated how self-serving passion could be if reason became its handmaiden.

The unbridled and indomitable exercise of will – 'iron will'– can lead to the worst kind of evil: we have already considered the Nazis who whole-heartedly and wilfully embraced a policy of German domination. Passion, too, can easily turn to selfishness and lead to another kind of exploitation of others, although, because it so consumes the mind, it rarely leads to the kind of systematic evil that will can.

Imposing one's will or gratifying one's passion is usually at the expense of others. So, although it may lead to a kind of life satisfaction, it cannot lead to well-being for the reasons that we argued in the last chapter. Something must curb the will and control passion – or so it seems. Values are one means of doing this: as they counteract the excitement of letting oneself go with negative feelings of disgust or anxiety. Values create habits. Aristotle thought that habitual self-control changed the direction of the will. Hume thought that passions schooled by one's mother became habitual as well.

Sartre (1969), though, rejected values or habits imposed by other people, because he thought that they were self-inflicted privations that reduced a person's freedom. This does seem to create the very situation of licence and licentiousness that his critics taxed him with.

Where do we find self-control?

Neuropsychologists have recently returned to what has been an old-fashioned idea for a long time – self-control. It is a bit of a paradoxical idea, too, if we assume as we did in the previous section that we rely on others to control us, either directly or through the shaming that Sartre described so vividly in his account of the gaze (Sartre, 1969). In one study of 1000 people, followed up from birth to the age of 32 , self-control in children was associated with better physical health, less substance dependence, better personal finances and less criminal offending outcomes in adults (Moffitt et al., 2011). In a further study of another 500 children who each had one sibling with lower self-control, the less self-controlled sibling had a worse outcome as an adult (Moffitt et al., 2011).

Self-control in children might be a proxy for social control, but the sibling element of the Moffitt et al. study suggests that the outcomes could not simply be put down to parenting (although parents do not always treat each child the same, so sibling controls are never fully satisfactory). Something in the child made the difference. One commonly suggested candidate for this something is delayed gratification: the willingness to put off an immediate reward if a bigger one could be obtained later. Delayed gratification has also been associated with better health, such as a more normal weight (Seeyave et al., 2009), higher income and greater happiness in later life. It is fostered by thinking about the future (Cheng et al., 2012) and it would not stretch the imagination too far to call it 'vision'.

Sartre, too, repeatedly considers the influence of vision over our lives. Not that he thinks we can see our goal, but we can look along the likely course of our future path – which he calls, the project – and imagine where it might take us if we continue along that route.

Looking ahead

Looking ahead is a common theme for many of the philosophers, psychologists, economists and others that we have considered in this chapter. What is unique about Sartre, and we think is more like the human condition, is that we look out from multiple viewpoints (unless we allow ourselves to be fixed by the gaze of another to be looking always through the same keyhole) and when we look, we do not see a goal or look towards a goal we know to be there. We can look only a short way: not enough to see where the path ends, but enough to ask ourselves, is this my path? Do I want to go this way?

This still leaves open the question of whether or not I want to go forward in that way, and here I think that passion and values do come into it: not as determinants of the choice, but as determinants of the atmosphere in which the choice is made. Perhaps I see that my path will lead me to fighting and possible death, or to conflict and possible abandonment. Even contemplating the vision will arouse passionate feelings, both for and against. Passion *for* might come from a rage at injustice and a passion to put it right, but it will often be counter-balanced by fear and disgust at the possibility of bodily injury. Other people's values will determine their reactions to my choices and contribute to the emotional atmosphere. If I am an adolescent deciding to stand up to punitive parents, I am likely to get support from other adolescents who value autonomy and independence, but criticism from my parents' peers who will condemn me if they are children of the book for breaking the fifth commandment (its equivalent is in surah 17 in the Qu'ran).

Our dispositions are expressed in our actions, but particularly in this instance in where we look and what we see. These dispositions are also changed by the consequences of our actions. We find out about them through reflecting on our actions too. As Aristotle suggested, we can sometimes use this to consciously alter our actions and reactions so that our habitual dispositions gradually change. Passion and values are prudential guides, but do not have to be the determinants of our actions unless we stumble blindly forward in our life.

Control over our well-being is limited by external circumstances, genetics and all of the other influences that we have considered so far. But we do have some control over it and we have already considered that. We can influence our health through diet, exercise and our use of intoxicants. We can influence our well-being through maintaining good relationships, dealing effectively with conflicts and making the most of our opportunities to earn a comfortable income whilst not becoming addicted to money-making.

Life satisfaction is greatest if our projects succeed, but we have been arguing in this chapter that our projects, in Sartre's sense, cannot be pre-planned. So the best that we can do to achieve life satisfaction is to widen and deepen our vision whilst being open to the influence of, but not being driven by, our values and our passions.

How do we widen our vision? Multiple perspectives are important, that is being able to see things from several different points of view, including the different points of view of different people. It also means being able to see deeply into things, which implies not being caught up in one aspect or another of the total panorama and getting good at interpreting signs or portents.

When passion defeats vision

Sometimes passion, extreme demanding emotion, takes over even if we have been able to live a balanced, prudential life (although it is much more likely to take over if we have not). Vision is no longer needed in this situation. We proceed using our proximal senses of touch and smell, and as these senses are so closely linked to taste, we react with hunger or desire, or nausea and disgust. Sooner or later, these emotions abate and we often find that we have stumbled into a new present, with a quite different future. We may have tried to look ahead even at the height of our passion, but probably not for long and not with any real confidence that we would want to see where we were going. At a certain point, we do want to see the way ahead again, and it may be that the way seems too difficult. We may find ourselves with financial problems; alienated from friends and family; reputationally damaged; or feeling that the future will take us further and further away from our previous sense of security.

A long-term and thriving future is often hardly visible in this situation, as our path has to skirt around so many obstacles and so many pitfalls that we cannot see where it goes, or indeed whether it goes anywhere. The English word for this kind of narrow, perhaps blocked, path is 'straits': hence the expression being in 'dire straits'. One Latin translation for 'straits' is 'angustiae', meaning narrow or straitened, but itself derived from the verb angustere, meaning to throttle or choke. Many of the terms for anxiety (including anxiety itself, angst, anguish, anxieux in French and angusta in Spanish) in modern European languages come from angustere.

Narrowing down our vision is accompanied by anxiety and a fear of being choked off. It is tempting to turn our eyes away in response to this level of anxiety and go backwards rather than forwards. This of course makes all of the actions that we have taken motivated by passion, pointless. It is not that the passion was wrong – passions cannot in themselves be right or wrong, only unfeigned and genuine or illusory – but by failing to follow through on the path into which our passion was projected, we dissociated ourselves from taking responsibility for its consequences and so made the passion destructive. The only justification for acting passionately rather than rationally is if we are prepared to follow through with our reason to live as well as we can with the consequences of our passionate actions.

Glamour

To be described as grammared has not always been without its downside. Reading and writing have sometimes seemed magical in the bad sense of putting a spell on people. The French word for a book of spells – 'grimoire' – is derived from the French for grammar, 'grammaire' or in Scots, 'grammarye'. In Scots, 'grammarye' also had a magical connotation, with this meaning of enchantment becoming strengthened as the word was transmuted to 'glamour'. It was often used of gypsies or card-sharps who had an uncanny power to deceive. Robert Burns included this line in one of his poems: 'Ye gipsy-gang that deal in glamor, And you, deep-read in hell's black grammar, Warlocks and witches' (*Poems*: II. 220).

It was in this sense, of casting a glamour over someone or something, that it was popularized in English by Sir Walter Scott in his *Letters on Demonology* (Scott, 1884). Glamour has lost its unwelcome, diabolical associations since the 1840s when Scott was writing. The enchantment is now wholly welcome, and indeed it seems to be what men expect of women who can be complimented by being called 'glamorous', as well as enchanting, spell-binding, captivating or arresting.

All of these words refer to a state that would normally be unwelcome, often shaming, but becomes desirable when combined with something highly desired. The deception is so attractive that we return to it voluntarily, in an act of self-deception. This explains why confidence tricksters, another group who cast a glamour, do not always leave their victims angry when they are exposed. Some victims want to continue to believe. They prefer the glamour to the reality. They are prepared to prolong deception as self-deception. Effective confidence tricksters start by offering something that another person desires. The 'bait' may be sex or money or even something very simple like finding an apparently thrown away thumb-stick (Wilhelm & Andress, 2011). Whatever it is, it becomes enchanting if it takes a person out of their everyday world into a new, absorbing one, in which desires are satisfied and wishes granted without any of the disappointments that we have seen in earlier chapters.

People who use drugs, pornography, fetishism, gambling or other 'addictive' states often secretly believe, like people who are conned, that the meretricious happiness associated with the first exposure to these activities could actually provide them with well-being. Child abusers convince themselves that not only they, but the children who are abused, are somehow in a better world. Drug users believe that they see more of reality than those who abstain. It is obvious to other people that they are deluded, but are they more deluded than, say, a scientist who spends her whole life on jungle expeditions to study a rare primate, or an artist like Van Gogh who only comes alive when painting? What is the difference?

One kind of answer is that the former are not living in reality – they are not 'reality-testing', to use a word from psychoanalytic psychotherapy. We have learnt, partly through Sartre himself, to distrust this claim, however. One person's reality may not be another's. But there is still some force to the claim. The person who lives in an enchanted world can tolerate all manner of relationship disrepair, environmental squalor, even poor health without noticing these realities. These unpleasant aspects of their life only become obvious when, as we say, 'the scales fall from their eyes' and they start to see clearly again. This might happen as the result of an injunction to 'look at yourself', but more often comes about because the effort to maintain the glamour becomes more and more onerous and life becomes proportionately less and less satisfying.

What do people do when the glamour wears off or when passion cools? These are often black moments, when our vision of our future fails. This does not mean that our mental 'vision' has failed, any more than our metaphor of vision means that people with visual impairment have less vision about their future than sighted people.

But our ability to pursue our vision may be limited by more than a lack of courage or the fear that our vision is pointing us to try something that is impossible. We may sometimes be held back from taking action by something that is pulling us in a different direction or is paralysing us. We may be held back by our fear of being criticized or shamed, and we may be paralysed by feeling that we do not even know what path we are meant to follow.

One way that people may think of this is that their world has changed and the roads they once knew are no longer there. The old signs and way markers no longer mean what they did: there is a 'meaning vacuum'.

The meaning vacuum

'Waking up' to one's true situation, when an enchantment is broken, when one stops deceiving oneself, or when passion becomes questionable, is like finding oneself in a new and uncanny world. A catastrophic life event often has a similar effect. It is like starting over as a child, but as a child we are gradually inculcated into the world and may never experience that sense of aimlessness or emptiness associated with the 'new world' experience. Some people do experience it in adolescence, when they leave home or when they realize that life is taking them beyond the limits of their parents' understanding.

In a new world like this, old signposts may no longer work. We cannot, for example, aim along our path as we had previously done. At first, we may be locked in by negative emotions, and, like a wounded animal for whom every movement is a fresh pain, we may just want to curl up and avoid any but the most survival-orientated actions. But even when our passions are no longer locked in negative mode, there may seem to be no point in acting, because whether we do or we don't it has no meaning. Sometimes, there is meaning, but only in the past. So our whole concern is to try to keep the past alive, a reaction sometimes to bereavement in which the dead person is kept alive as a kind of hidden presence, but the same process also applies to people who undertake extended litigation or appeals about losing a job or money, not because they want justice but because they want to put off the day when they have to accept that the job or the money has finally gone.

As I noted in the previous chapter, meaning making is linked very closely with well-being. A world that is meaningless is rarely a world that affords its inhabitants happiness. Meaning of life is linked to health, too, such as in lengthening survival in women with breast cancer (Neyt & Albrecht, 2006).

Aristotle, whose guidance I have fallen back on so often, did not consider this situation. The practical wisdom that he suggested should be the guide to well-being was developed in relation to a particular class of aristocrats in a moment of stability in the Greek world. At the time that he wrote, his pupil Alexander was destroying the Iranian empire, it is said with Aristotle's encouragement, but Thessaloniki, near where Aristotle was brought up, and Athens, where Aristotle's academy was founded, were thriving and peaceful. Aristotle's ethics applies to autonomous, well-off and well-respected people like him (and one cannot help thinking, like many proponents of positive psychology). It does not provide guidance when the world collapses. The Stoics, who applied Aristotle's ideas about virtue did consider catastrophe (one of its founders, Epictetus, was a freed slave), but, like the Epicureans, took the view that one should be content with very little and not expect much more satisfaction in life than a righteous sense of being virtuous. If a person no longer had the means to live well, the Stoics, like Seneca who opened his veins in a bath rather than continue to advise Nero, thought that suicide was justified.

Suicide suits tyrants well. It relieves them of a thorn in their side. Suicide also leaves other people bereft and let down. Stoicism did not take account of the connectedness of people to each other, but focused on an individual living well. However, as we saw in the last chapter, living well cannot ignore our influence on other people and their influence on us.

Connectedness and meaning are interwoven. When confronted with a changed world, the first thing we do is try to find connections between it and our old one. Connections enable us to come up with explanations, and therefore gain mastery, and this is especially important when we are least secure, as we are when we contemplate choices about our futures. Anything is grist for connecting, hence the proliferation of half-baked theories about destiny. One of these, nominative determinism, gives a good illustration of the glamour that oracular theories have. An example is given on the website 'Quirkology' by Professor Wiseman (an example itself perhaps of nominative determinism, unless he changed his name by deed poll) of the Bulgarian hurdler who fell in her 400m qualifying heat at the London Olympics in 2012. Her name was Stambolova. Plenty of the commentators on this example were unimpressed: 'Did she know enough English to appreciate how her name might be read by English people?' was one such comment.

Half-baked, we said, about such theories but connections do subtly influence us. There has been one serious statistically sophisticated study suggesting that nominative determinism may influence life decisions (Pelham et al., 2002).

We do not really think that there is a causal connection between Miss Stambolova's last name and her failure to qualify for the final in London. But we do think that the lure of nominative determinism, even to very rational people, is its ability to link events within a larger context of meaning. Dreams, stories, dance and film all create a skein of meaning, linking disparate events in a mesh work of meaning. One function of this is to absorb purely contingent or unmotivated events, and restore a sense of predictability and mastery on which meaning relies.

The interconnection of facts, names, experiences, people and any other emotionally flavoured elements is a key contributor to meaning, but the connections must carry an emotional charge for us to feel that they are 'meaningful'. Nominative determinism carries such a charge because it carries away our anxiety about the future.

One meaning leads to another, but if one of the linked meanings becomes dangerously negative, the interconnection breaks down, and so does the capacity to make meaning out of experience or, as people actually experience it, meaning it disappears from experience leaving a vacuum.

This existential vacuum is a common consequence of catastrophe of all kinds. It is a consequence of passion, too, although this is less recognized, for passion also encourages us – sometimes even forces us – to exchange our old but accustomed world for a new, strange and risky one. For a while, the passion itself sustains us, but there comes a moment when that stops being enough: we find ourselves in a comparable vacuum of meaning.

Living well/the good life

Living well or living the good life often mean living comfortably, sometimes with an implication that one is living more comfortably than one's neighbours. Living high on the hog is another phrase with a similar meaning, and it is tempting, sometimes, not to echo Einstein's sentiment that to live this way is a bit swinish.

In the last section of this chapter, I shall consider what the 'good life' means in the sense that is used of another person – that they did not just live a good life, but were a good person too. Living a good life is not easy. It presupposes, for one thing, that one knows what 'the good' is.

Psychotherapists often deal with people who feel that they are in a moral vacuum which is gradually extinguishing their life. Two questions often come up: 'Did I do wrong?' and 'What should I do to be a good person?'

Neither has an answer and yet both must be answered if the therapy is to be successful. The first question is one we have already considered. Some acts are wrong according to law or custom, but people do not ask psychotherapists whether these are right or wrong – they already know. The question more often means, 'Am I forgiven?' or 'What will people think of me?' In fact, it's not such a different question from, 'What should I do?' which often comes down to, 'If I do what I want to do, or am tempted to do, what will people think of me?', sometimes with the rider, 'and will they forgive me?'

Unusually at these moments, we have the opportunity to decide on living well or not. Conventional wisdom is that we choose the religiously or morally sanctioned option, or we do what someone we respect would do, or we do what would be least harmful to other people. In this chapter, I have argued that to choose as others would might fall short of living well if, as I believe, living well means to fulfil one's potential for well-being and life satisfaction. Of course, the impact on other people cannot be discounted. I argued in the last chapter that a fully developed human being has a fully developed empathic connection with others (an interbrain connection, as we called it) that means that other people's suffering is contagious, particularly if that suffering is caused by us.

Obeying the rules because they are rules is not living up to our full potential. We have to choose to obey the rules. Living well often means choosing to obey rules, but we cannot rely on the rules to tell us what to do if we want to live as well as we can. For that, we have to make a choice we can live with and make good on, for us and for other people. So the answer to the question, 'Did I do right or wrong?' is itself a question: 'Are you determined to make what you did turn out right – or as right as it can be – for all concerned?' and the answer to 'What should I do?', or at least the answer from the perspective of enhancing well-being, is: 'Think of your various possible courses of action, and consider which one will lead to the greatest enhancement of your life satisfaction, with the greatest possibility of you being able to enhance the life satisfaction of those others who are affected by your decision'.

Connectedness

A key feature of all theories of the good is that they take account of connectedness with other people. We overlook the vagaries of the privately immoral behaviour of our favoured artists if their art adds enough that is positive to our lives. Artists have the capacity to connect with thousands, if not millions, of others although each individual connection is weak. For the rest of us, the main recipients of our good, or our evil, are those with whom we connect more intimately and therefore more strongly. Whether our life increases their well-being and therefore their potential for life satisfaction is one of the main determinants, in my view, of how well or badly we have lived.

10

Applied Well-being

Good health and happiness are so closely interlinked as to be effectively two sides of the same coin, which I have called 'well-being'. Well-being does not often show itself through our feelings: only exceptionally do we feel a healthy glow or a joyful rush. Artificially producing these states, for example by drugs, often reduces well-being in the long run. So aiming for euphoria is not, according to almost every philosopher, the best way to increase our well-being. So how do we do this? We are fortunate if we live in a community where tradition dictates a healthy lifestyle, and if our mental and social capital is high so that we adopt the tradition whole-heartedly. If we cannot rely on tradition, we must fall back on science. Either way, maintaining or improving well-being tends to be a deliberate activity. We can, for example, learn what diet increases longevity, and adopt that; or make an effort to keep up our fitness by walking rather than taking the bus or just staying at home. Positive psychologists have comparable strategies to increase our positive feelings and couples counsellors give advice about maintaining positive relationships. Many of these strategies have been covered in previous chapters.

Life would be easy if we all had control over the direction of our lives, freedom from conflict or want to ruffle its surface, a good genetic stock giving us a positive hedonic balance and no genes for disease or premature old age, and reciprocated loving relationships with others. Our conscious efforts to improve our well-being could be exercised fully, without any of the ennervating effects of negative feelings or negative events, but fortunately life is rarely this easy. Fortunately, because life satisfaction is often linked to the effort that we have to put into gaining well-being rather than just having it dropped in our lap. Life satisfaction is more closely linked to life expectancy in people than well-being (Strobel et al., 2011), a particular that may be uniquely human. Health and happiness are directly correlated with life expectancy in orang-utans (Weiss et al., 2011).

One of the reasons that feelings are not an ideal predictor of life expectancy is that most people live for more than having good feelings. They also live to realize their goals. Defining what these goals are is often difficult, but many people believe that they cannot just be concerned with their own welfare. There has to be something beyond this, something transcendent. This is often provided for by spiritual beliefs – in the family, in religion, in nature, in work or in social improvement. Sometimes, something happens to make these goals seem absurd. This 'existential crisis' may plunge a person into depression, with the effect of shortening their life and destroying their happiness. Or it may lead to what Kierkegaard called a 'leap of faith' onto a new path. The difficulty is that we may not know where this path leads, until we get there. I argued in the previous chapter that the only way to deal with this is to stick to your path courageously once it has been chosen.

The other challenge to taking a completely new path in life is that it disturbs not only our own equilibrium, but also that of other people. We cannot just ignore this. People, unlike solitary orang-utans, cannot help but live for others. That is why the two expressions, 'I always try to have a good time' and 'I always try to live a good life' are so similar and yet so different. Having a good time often implies 'irrespective of how other people are feeling', yet it is impossible to live a good life without taking other people's feelings into account. I have used, and will continue in this chapter to use, 'living well' in this extended sense – to mean more than 'I live well, I've got a good income'; something more like, 'He lived well, and we should all celebrate what his life has meant to us'.

Living well is not just about feelings. I have also argued that many people live to accomplish goals or aims as well, even if determining what these are may sometimes only be possible in hindsight. Accomplishing these goals, or even getting near them, is a source of cognitive reward, for which I have generally used the term life satisfaction. Living well involves living a satisfying life, and this usually means a life in which there have been times of doubt, uncertainty or fear, disappointment, and so on. It may have also meant not living up to other people's expectations, but cleaving to one's own. So living well has to be tempered by living a satisfying life: there is a cognitive element of accomplishment as well as an affective element of positivity.

In this last chapter, I will consider one of the last remaining problems raised in Chapter 1. Sartre (1969) was once challenged to say how his idea that a person who did not live in freedom was living in bad faith might apply to a prisoner. Aristotle admitted that his ideas about happiness could not apply to those who did not have freedom, which included the slaves who made sure that Aristotle had the freedom from daily chores to write philosophy. Aristotle also thought that people who were ill or who had chronic family problems could never achieve full life satisfaction. How do we account for people who may not be able to escape limitations on their well-being? Can they achieve life satisfaction and live well?

What limitations are there on well-being?

Happiness is, as we have seen, influenced by early life experience and by genetics. Health may be affected by chronic disease developing at any age, or by the risk of being exposed to virulent infectious disease. The power to change one's life is necessary for life satisfaction, but not everyone has that power. Relationships can destroy as well as heal. Want, lack of shelter, exposure to war or other conflicts, and crime: these can all reduce the quality of life.

Should we alter our conceptions of living well for different groups of people whose lives are affected by some of these limiting factors, or should we consider, like Aristotle, that they simply cannot live well and there is nothing we can do? Health economists routinely rate one person's year of life as being of lower quality than another. Does this mean that one person has more quality than another, and that, for example, more resources should go to the higher quality person than the lower quality one? There is a persistent idea, which resurfaces on a regular basis, that some people are more deserving of life than others. Does the quality of life argument support this? If it is the case that circumstances restrict the well-being of some people compared to others – for example, through infectious disease, disability or mere want – should these people's lives be discounted compared to those with more well-being? Is the extravert worth more than the introvert? I shall try to consider some of these unpleasant, hardly to be thought of, questions before ending this chapter and the book.

Want

Many people in the West apologize for spending so much time talking about psychological well-being when so many people in the world are starving. They presume that unhappiness is a lesser evil, has a lesser impact on well-being than, say, hunger. Psychotherapists often attribute this 'truth' to Maslow, who propounded a hierarchy of human needs (Maslow, 1968), and the doctrine that until basic needs are met 'higher' needs are of no concern.

Empirical findings do not support this. Hunger is often associated with an increase in health in previously affluent societies. In the Cienfuegos province of Cuba, for example, in the years following the special period of severe shortage of food and fuel, there was a fall in obesity, in diabetes and in diabetes-related mortality (Franco et al., 2013). In another large study, positive and negative emotions were more strongly associated with self-reported health than hunger, homelessness and threats to security (Pressman et al., 2013).

Acceptance of the Maslovian hierarchy of needs may reflect Western prejudices about people in other, less developed parts of the world, much as European psychiatrists in Africa once assumed that native Africans did not experience depression because they were too concerned with survival.

Life can be satisfying even in the presence of want, just as life can be unsatisfying in the presence of plenty. Perhaps we are wrong to ignore satisfaction when we give people aid to recover from disasters. For disasters bring not just want and disease but the vitiation of former life goals, with their victims struggling to find a new path in life.

The case of autism

Barnbaum (2008) argues that if there were a cure for autism, people would not choose to take it, and nor would it be ethical to apply it. This is despite the considerable difficulties that many people with autism have. She argues that this is because people with autism have 'integrity'. Russell (2012), a bioethicist, disagrees. She identifies three main ways that integrity is defined by moral philosophers: (1) as 'an uncompromising commitment to honour certain laudable values, including oral, spiritual and aesthetic ones' (p. 166); (2) having a lively sense of what is right by other people, and putting aside one's own habits and preferences in order to do what is right by others; and (3) being consistent in one's emotional responses, beliefs and values. Russell argues that people with an autism spectrum disorder (ASD) cannot, because of what she takes to be their impairments, demonstrate integrity on any of these criteria.

Russell's (2012) argument seems to me to hold good for her second and third definitions of integrity, but not for the first. She argues that the first kind of integrity, 'an uncompromising commitment to honour certain values', arises in people who want to be thought of by others as 'honest', but since people with an ASD may not be motivated by a wish to gain the approval of others (she terms these 'second-order desires') then they are not likely to be honest. I would imagine that anyone who knows people with an ASD would be surprised at this conclusion. Certainly I know that I am. 'Honesty' might be the middle name of most people with an ASD, and if they had two middle names the second might be 'uncompromising'. I would say, contra Russell, that it is the fact that people with an ASD combine a disinterest in, or really an unawareness of, other people's opinions with honesty that gives them a higher degree of integrity than neurotypicals. They just are as they are, irrespective of the situation, the company or their own interests.

'Integrity' is only a virtue if it is a feature of intention. It cannot be applied to people with ASD, with severe intellectual disability and no usable language or speech, or indeed anyone with this degree of intellectual disability. Does that mean we should not concern ourselves with the life satisfaction of people with severe developmental disabilities, just as in orphanages and institutions their well-being has easily been sacrificed on many occasions.

Implications for applied well-being

Whether or not a person with an ASD is recognized as having integrity or not has implications for their well-being. It is true that few people with an ASD would promote themselves, and so it might seem that they are unconcerned about others' evaluation of them, but granting a person with ASD integrity is granting them a valued place in society.

My treatment of well-being in earlier chapters has focused on a person's ability to achieve well-being without taking account of other people's ability to deprive a person of well-being. No argument is needed to establish that one person can deprive another of happiness, or health. The fact is conceded in law, which considers that both acts are punishable crimes. But depriving someone of life satisfaction is not necessarily a crime, and yet it may prevent them from living as well as they might otherwise have done.

Many people who are different in some way that society finds challenging experience bullying: 9 out of 10 people with Asperger's syndrome, a form of ASD, said that they have or are still being bullied in one study (Balfe & Tantam, 2010). Bullying may induce long-term negative feelings, and therefore poor health, but at least most people would consider it wrong. Blocking someone's ability to live well is more subtle and less obvious.

The academic discussion between Russell and Barnbaum seems just that, an academic discussion. But one of its consequences – were it to become widely accepted anyway – is whether or not a person with an ASD could exemplify an accepted virtue and, in so doing, live well. There are other examples of life principles that could be taken to be virtuous or dismissed as being the empty simulacra of virtue: courage or thoughtless persistence; humility or subservience; kindness or needing to be liked.

If readers agree that living well must take account, as Bentham and Comte argued, of others, then living well would seem to require giving other people respect and recognition of their virtues even if, or perhaps especially if, these other people are individuals who are disadvantaged, unhealthy or unhappy.

Well-being and aging

The same considerations apply to people with dementia, who have deteriorated to the point where it is impossible to know how much they are aware of their circumstances. There has been a strong focus on 'good aging' where high self-esteem, resilience and physical fitness combine to make aging a satisfying experience (Tumminello et al., 2011). But what about 'less good' aging? Can anyone take satisfaction in that, or is dementia, like intellectual disability, a bar to life satisfaction?

Clearly, no one can be satisfied that dementia, microcephaly and other disabilities reduce some people's quality of life. It is right that researchers should try to ameliorate or prevent these conditions. But it seems to me that it would be wrong to infer from this that a demented person's life is unsatisfactory, even if we can be fairly sure that they lack the capacity to reflect on their life and make the judgement themselves.

The eudaimonic unit

Aristotle's famous *Nicomachean Ethics* amounted to advice for an Athenian citizen. I have noted that this limits its applicability, but not considered what the ideal scope of a similar ethical document might be. One obvious starting point is that it should be ethical advice for any person, but that begs a definition of 'person'. One way around this is to take 'person' as a given, as what other persons treat as being a person. Obviously, the actual scope of this might change from being a person in a smaller group than the collectivity of living organisms with human DNA (consider foetuses or human cell line cultures) or in a larger group than that collectivity (consider corpses immediately after life has fled, pets and other great apes). If people are connected by empathic ties, then perhaps the unit of consideration for well-being and life satisfaction is not the individual but a group, or unit, of persons united by empathic ties. Aristotle refers to the ties of family in the *Nicomachean Ethics* but, as noted in Chapter 1, says that the boundaries of this unit of people are too diffuse to be able to deal with it and so ignores it. But the problem of deciding on the boundaries of a eudaimonic unit is one that each of us deals with constantly. Do I feel enough of a tie with these disaster victims to make a contribution? Am I close enough to that person to travel a long distance to attend their funeral? My second cousin wants to come and stay, but I am having a very busy week. Are they close enough family for me to be under an obligation to entertain them?

If it is the eudaimonic unit, and not the individual, that is the subject of the *Nicomachean Ethics*, then Aristotle's views on life satisfaction following from the practice of life skills can be applied to the unit, except that the skills are not about individual excellence but about the communitarian skills of living as a unit that encompass the person who may not be able to gain life satisfaction alone but is essential to the development of communitarian life skills such as care. These are not unfamiliar skills, since they are the virtues of collective cultures (Etzioni, 2012).

Some final conclusions

Whether or not a person has lived well is not a judgement that can be made by one person, not even by the person themselves. In taking this position, I am rejecting the authority of many religions that claim to be able to make these judgements, and I apologize to any reader who might be offended. However, as we are here in the realm of belief, I must state my own. I have met many people, and have read about even more, who I think have lived well. Some of them were religious, but certainly not all. I would not be able to say what it was about the pattern of their lives that I interpreted as living well and I conclude that there is no blueprint for living well, any more than there is for producing a great work of art. Even if there were such a blueprint, I can easily imagine a new way of living that does not fit the blueprint, but which I would want to call living well.

I will therefore end on a completely personal note: how I have applied the principles that I have been weighing up in this book in my own life.

I think that I can describe some things that would give me pause before accepting that someone had lived well. Harming, exploiting or just denying life satisfaction to other people would be included in my list, for example. However, causing other people to be harmed cannot be a sufficient criterion for denying that a person has lived well, else soldiers, surgeons, judges and a whole range of other people would be ruled out. There are even more complex cases: Napoleon, Alexander, Mao Zedong and other figures who changed history. Did they live well? They certainly caused the deaths of hundreds of thousands, even millions, of people.

Most people would say that Hitler did not live well, but Roosevelt did. Both committed their respective countries to war, and so initiated the killing of many hundreds of thousands of people. Both claimed to be doing this in the interests of their country, but Hitler thought it right to kill the disabled, the mentally ill, the Rom, the Jews, the Slavs as well as the enemy. Hitler took much more in his avowed aim to give to his country than Roosevelt. In fact, he took so much that the taking of life, the extermination process itself, became an end rather than a means. So living well includes a positive element of what a person makes of their life, and a negative element, what they take from life in order to achieve it. It is a necessary criterion of living well that the making has to outweigh the taking. Taking does not only mean the taking of life, but the taking of security, trust or the environment, and readers will have their own items to add to this list.

Life satisfaction is not a public judgement, but purely a subjective one, unlike living well. However, they are clearly linked. A person who thought that they had lived well is also likely to be satisfied with their life, but many people may feel that they cannot know that they have lived well, although they may say that they tried to. Being satisfied with one's life is a judgement. Like any judgement, it may be poor, a misjudgement. When it is a judgement about oneself, a degree of self-deception is likely to be involved. Self-deception was considered as one kind of 'incontinence', or an inability to act on intentions and plans. I argued in that chapter (Chapter 7) that acting on plans often requires using a resource, just like living well, although in this case the resource is personal. It has appeared throughout the book, although referred to in different words: reward, in the early chapters, persistence, grip, determination, executive function and self-regulation. Contributions to each of these are made by well-being, in that happy, healthy people are more likely to be able to persevere, but what Aristotle and many others since have called 'character' is also a factor. Aristotle argued that these virtues or strengths can be further strengthened by practice, and this may be true, although recent evidence suggests that acting in a righteous way on one occasion is more, not less, likely to lead to backsliding on the next.

As for living well, it might be more illuminating to look at what detracts from virtue as what makes for it. Defeat obviously does. In a world where virtue is punished, virtue does not survive for long. Bullying, abuse, conflictual or unsatisfying relationships, opportunities snatched away, bad luck, rotten job, good job but with pay far inferior to the neighbours, criminal convictions – all of these humdrum but ennervating circumstances can sap the virtue to make good on life satisfaction. Trying to deal with this by taking more than life can give makes the situation worse. Taking more in this case means believing in magic to make the situation right, or dwelling on the past to find some way of changing it, or offering up suffering as a justification for pursuing self-defeat because it is the least demanding path, which it usually is.

Giving positive definitions is never as easy as listing exceptions, but I would agree with Aristotle that happiness and health are excellences. By this I mean that they are states of being which require effort or skill on our part to achieve and to maintain and which we can never fully reach. They are clearly closely related excellences too. Happy people tend to be healthier, and healthy people tend to be happier, so a compound excellence, that I have termed well-being in this book, makes sense.

Well-being is not so closely linked to life satisfaction, and may not be linked to living well at all. A person who suffers from a chronic disorder may have reduced well-being, but may have considerable life satisfaction (although that would require more than average fortitude). Similarly, a person who lives in dangerous or dispiriting circumstances, and faces up to these even though they may become fearful or low in consequence, may have considerable life satisfaction in knowing that they have been honest and avoided self-deception.

Most of us would disagree with Aristotle's absolutist approach to excellence. He was asked whether a man being racked could be happy, and if so, whether that man could be virtuous. He thought not. But surely a man who has been racked who can survive with an unbroken spirit, or a woman who has had a traumatic childbirth who can still look with love on her child, have a kind of excellence too.

This kind of excellence is not about achieving a limit but about approximating another kind of limit, of the requirements of others. The person who shows fortitude in the face of terrible pain is also making no claim for comfort or protection; no demand that they should be spared. The person whose happiness comes through the sacrifice or abuse of others is making very large claims on the world. That person is making a big withdrawal on the well-being capital of the world. These withdrawals do not just involve claims on people. They may be claims on the environment that provides life satisfaction to others, or even claims on a person's own body.

Excellence and claims, investments and withdrawals, both need to be counted but they are not amounts of fixed value like money; rather, their value varies according to our own reckoning. Bentham's (1876) felicific calculus works over populations as he intended where a common value can be applied, but it relies too heavily on feelings as accurate indicators of investment and withdrawal. Pain may trigger a withdrawal and pleasure enable an investment but feelings are not synonymous with states. Nor can one balance one's account, and decide on that basis whether one is living well or not, or even whether one should be satisfied with one's life or not.

Whether we have lived well or ill is something that we will discover only in retrospect, or perhaps even not then, since it is ultimately a judgement for others to make. Whether it's even worth trying for can be doubted. For me, it is difficult to see why else one would live at all.

References

Abel, T., & Frohlich, K. L. (2012). Capitals and capabilities: linking structure and agency to reduce health inequalities. *Social Science & Medicine, 74*(2), 236–244. doi: 10.1016/j.socscimed.2011.10.028

Adam, E. K., Gunnar, M. R., & Tanaka, A. (2004). Adult attachment, parent emotion, and observed parenting behavior: mediator and moderator models. *Child Development, 75*(1), 110–122.

Adolphs, R., Gosselin, F., Buchanan, T. W., Tranel, D., Schyns, P., & Damasio, A. R. (2005). A mechanism for impaired fear recognition after amygdala damage. *Nature, 433*(7021), 68–72.

Ajzen, I., & Madden, T. (1986). Prediction of goal-directed behavior: attitudes, intentions and perceived behavioral control. *Journal of Experimental and Social Psychology, 22*, 453–474.

Akresh, R., Lucchetti, L., & Thirumurthy, H. (2012). Wars and child health: evidence from the Eritrean–Ethiopian conflict. *Journal of Development Economics, 99*(2), 330–340. doi: 10.1016/j.jdeveco.2012.04.001

Alex Linley, P., Maltby, J., Wood, A. M., Joseph, S., Harrington, S., Peterson, C., . . . Seligman, M. E. P. (2007). Character strengths in the United Kingdom: the VIA Inventory of Strengths. *Personality and Individual Differences, 43*(2), 341–351. doi: http://dx.doi.org/10.1016/j.paid.2006.12.004

Ali, F., & Chamorro-Premuzic, T. (2010). The dark side of love and life satisfaction: associations with intimate relationships, psychopathy and Machiavellianism. *Personality and Individual Differences, 48*(2), 228–233. doi: http://dx.doi.org/10.1016/j.paid.2009.10.016

Allchin, A. M. (1997). *N. F. S. Grundtvig: an introduction to his life and work*. London: Darton, Longman, and Todd.

Ando, M., Morita, T., Akechi, T., & Takashi, K. (2012). Factors in narratives to questions in the short-term life review interviews of terminally ill cancer patients and utility of the questions. *Palliative & Supportive Care*, 1–8. doi: 10.1017/S1478951511000708

Appiah, K. (2008). *Experiments in ethics*. Cambridge, MA: Harvard University Press.

Augustine, A. A., & Hemenover, S. H. (2008). Extraversion and the consequences of social interaction on affect repair. *Personality and Individual Differences, 44*(5), 1151–1161. doi: http://dx.doi.org/10.1016/j.paid.2007.11.009

Austin, N. (2010). Homeric nostalgia. *The Yale Review, 98*(2), 37–64. doi: 10.1111/j.1467-9736.2010.00598.x

Baaz, M. E., & Stern, M. (2009). Why do soldiers rape? Masculinity, violence, and sexuality in the armed forces in the Congo (DRC). *International Studies Quarterly, 53*(2), 495–518.

Balfe, M., & Tantam, D. (2010). A descriptive social and health profile of a community sample of adults and adolescents with Asperger syndrome. *BMC Research Notes, 3*(1), 300.

Barger, S., Donoho, C., & Wayment, H. (2009). The relative contributions of race/ethnicity, socioeconomic status, health, and social relationships to life satisfaction in the United States. *Quality of Life Research, 18*(2), 179–189. doi: 10.1007/s11136-008-9426-2

Barnbaum, D. R. (2008). *The ethics of autism: among them, but not of them*. Bloomington, IN: Indiana University Press.

Bartels, D. M., & Pizarro, D. A. (2011). The mismeasure of morals: antisocial personality traits predict utilitarian responses to moral dilemmas. *Cognition, 121*(1), 154–161. doi: http://dx.doi.org/10.1016/j.cognition.2011.05.010

Bartz, J. A., Zaki, J., Ochsner, K. N., Bolger, N., Kolevzon, A., Ludwig, N., & Lydon, J. E. (2010). Effects of oxytocin on recollections of maternal care and closeness. *Proceedings of the National Academy of Sciences*. doi: 10.1073/pnas.1012669107

Batcho, K. I. (2007). Nostalgia and the emotional tone and content of song lyrics. *The American Journal of Psychology, 120*(3), 361–381.

Baumeister, R. F., Bratslavsky, E., Muraven, M., & Tice, D. M. (1998). Ego depletion: is the active self a limited resource? *Journal of Personality and Social Psychology, 74*(5), 1252–1265.

Beddington, J., Cooper, C. L., Field, J., Goswami, U., Huppert, F. A., Jenkins, R., . . . Thomas, S. M. (2008). The mental wealth of nations. *Nature, 455*(7216), 1057–1060.

BeDuhn, J. (2000). *The Manichaean body: in discipline and ritual*. Baltimore, MD: The Johns Hopkins University Press.

Beer, J. S. (2007). The default self: feeling good or being right? *Trends in Cognitive Sciences, 11*(5), 187–189. doi: 10.1016/j.tics.2007.02.004

Bellen, C. (2010). *Escapism and the restoration of the self: how terror management theory shakes consumption patterns*. Università della Svizzera Italiana.

Bennett, K. J., Torrance, G. W., Boyle, M. H., & Guscott, R. (2000). Cost-utility analysis in depression: the McSad utility measure for depression health states. *Psychiatr Serv, 51*(9), 1171–1176.

Bentham, J. (1876). *An introduction to the principles of morals and legislation*. Oxford: Clarendon Press.

Berrington de Gonzalez, A., Hartge, P., Cerhan, J. R., Flint, A. J., Hannan, L., MacInnis, R. J., . . . Thun, M. J. (2010). Body-Mass Index and mortality among 1.46 million white adults. *New England Journal Of Medicine, 363*(23), 2211–2219. doi: 10.1056/NEJMoa1000367

Bilder, R. M., & LeFever, F. F. (1998). *Neuroscience of the mind on the centennial of Freud's 'Project for a scientific psychology'*. New York: New York Academy of Sciences.

Blagosklonny, M. V. (2010). Why human lifespan is rapidly increasing: solving 'longevity riddle' with 'revealed-slow-aging' hypothesis. *Aging (Albany NY), 2*(4), 177–182.

Bonneux, L., Barendregt, J. J., Nusselder, W. J., & der Maas, P. J. (1998). Preventing fatal diseases increases healthcare costs: cause elimination life table approach [see comments]. *British Medical Journal, 316*(7124), 26–29.

Bossert, J. M., Stern, A. L., Theberge, F. R. M., Cifani, C., Koya, E., Hope, B. T., & Shaham, Y. (2011). Ventral medial prefrontal cortex neuronal ensembles mediate context-induced relapse to heroin. *Nature Neuroscience*, advance online publication: www.nature.com/neuro/journal/vaop/ncurrent/abs/nn.2758.html – supplementary-information

Bottan, N. L., & Perez Truglia, R. (2011). Deconstructing the hedonic treadmill: is happiness autoregressive? *Journal of Socio-Economics*, *40*(3), 224–236. doi: 10.1016/j.socec.2011.01.007

Brewer, J. A., Worhunsky, P. D., Gray, J. R., Tang, Y. Y., Weber, J., & Kober, H. (2011). Meditation experience is associated with differences in default mode network activity and connectivity. *Proceedings of the National Academy of Sciences of the United States of America*, *108*(50), 20254–20259. doi: 10.1073/pnas.1112029108

Brickman, P., & Campbell, D. (1971). Hedonic relativism and planning the good society. In M. Appley (Ed.), *Adaptation-level theory*. New York: Academic Press.

Brickman, P., Coates, D., & Janoff-Bulman, R. (1978). Lottery winners and accident victims: is happiness relative? *Journal of Personality and Social Psychology*, *36*(8), 917–927.

Brookings, J. B., & Serratelli, A. J. (2006). Positive illusions: positively correlated with subjective well-being, negatively correlated with a measure of personal growth. *Psychological Reports*, *98*(2), 407–413.

Burke, B. L., Martens, A., & Faucher, E. H. (2010). Two decades of terror management theory: a meta-analysis of mortality salience research. *Personality and Social Psychology Review*, *14*(2), 155–195.

Cacioppo, J. T., Hawkley, L. C., Norman, G. J., & Berntson, G. G. (2011). Social isolation. *Annals of the New York Academy of Sciences*, *1231*(1), 17–22. doi: 10.1111/j.1749-6632.2011.06028.x

Cahn, B. R., & Polich, J. (2006). Meditation states and traits: EEG, ERP, and neuroimaging studies. *Psychological Bulletin*, *132*(2), 180–211.

Cain, S. (2012). *Quiet: the power of introverts in a world that can't stop speaking.* Thorndike, ME: Center Point Pub.

Carrieri, V. (2012). Social comparison and subjective well-being: does the health of others matter? *Bulletin of Economic Research*, *64*(1), 31–55.

Carter, C. S. (2013). Oxytocin pathways and the evolution of human behavior. *Annual Review Of Psychology*. doi: 10.1146/annurev-psych-010213-115110

Cervinka, R., Roderer, K., & Hefler, E. (2012). Are nature lovers happy? On various indicators of well-being and connectedness with nature. *Journal of Health Psychology*, *17*(3), 379–388. doi: 10.1177/1359105311416873

Champagne, F., Diorio, J., Sharma, S., & Meaney, M. J. (2001). Naturally occurring variations in maternal behavior in the rat are associated with differences in estrogen-inducible central oxytocin receptors. *Proceedings of the National Academy of Sciences*, *98*(22), 12736.

Chaplin, L. N. (2009). Please may I have a bike? Better yet, may I have a hug? An examination of children's and adolescents' happiness. *Journal of Happiness Studies*, *10*(5), 541–562. doi: http://dx.doi.org/10.1007/s10902-008-9108-3

Chay, Y. W. (1993). Social support, individual differences and well-being: a study of small business entrepreneurs and employees. *Journal of Occupational and Organizational Psychology*, *66*(4), 285–302. doi: 10.1111/j.2044-8325.1993.tb00540.x

Cheng, J. T., Tracy, J. L., & Henrich, J. (2010). Pride, personality, and the evolutionary foundations of human social status. *Evolution and Human Behavior*, *31*(5), 334–347. doi: 10.1016/j.evolhumbehav.2010.02.004

Cheng, Y. Y., Shein, P. P., & Chiou, W. B. (2012). Escaping the impulse to immediate gratification: the prospect concept promotes a future-oriented mindset, prompting an inclination towards delayed gratification. *British Journal of Psychology*, *103*(1), 129–141. doi: 10.1111/j.2044-8295.2011.02067.x

Cherkas, L. F., Aviv, A., Valdes, A. M., Hunkin, J. L., Gardner, J. P., Surdulescu, G. L., . . . Spector, T. D. (2006). The effects of social status on biological aging as measured by white-blood-cell telomere length. *Aging Cell*, *5*(5), 361–365.

Chida, Y., Steptoe, A., & Powell, L. H. (2009). Religiosity/spirituality and mortality. *Psychotherapy And Psychosomatics*, *78*(2), 81–90.

Chilton, M., & Booth, S. (2007). Hunger of the body and hunger of the mind: African American women's perceptions of food insecurity, health and violence. *Journal of Nutrition Education and Behaviour*, *39*(3), 116–125. doi: 10.1016/j.jneb.2006.11.005

Chou, H. T., & Edge, N. (2012). 'They are happier and having better lives than I am': the impact of using Facebook on perceptions of others' lives. *Cyberpsychology, behavior and social networking*, *15*(2), 117–121. doi: 10.1089/cyber.2011.0324

Churchland, P. (1986). *Neurophilosophy: toward a unified science of the mind-brain*. Cambridge, MA: MIT Press.

Clark, H. C. (1994). *La Rochefoucauld and the language of unmasking in seventeenth-century France*. Geneva: Droz.

Cohen, S. (2004). Social relationships and health. *American Psychologist*, *59*(8), 676–684. doi: 10.1037/0003-066x.59.8.676

Cohn, M. A., Fredrickson, B. L., Brown, S. L., Mikels, J. A., & Conway, A. M. (2009). Happiness unpacked: positive emotions increase life satisfaction by building resilience. *Emotion*, *9*(3), 361–368. doi: 10.1037/a0015952

Colloca, L., & Miller, F. G. (2011). Harnessing the placebo effect: the need for translational research. *Philosophical Transactions of the Royal Society B: Biological Sciences*, *366*(1572), 1922–1930.

Connor-Smith, J. K., & Flachsbart, C. (2007). Relations between personality and coping: a meta-analysis. *Journal of Personality and Social Psychology*, *93*(6), 1080–1107. doi: 10.1037/0022-3514.93.6.1080

Courtois, S. P., & Kramer, M. (1999). *The black book of communism: crimes, terror, repression*. Cambridge, MA: Harvard University Press.

Crane, C., Jandric, D., Barnhofer, T., & Williams, J. M. (2010). Dispositional mindfulness, meditation, and conditional goal setting. *Mindfulness*, *1*(4), 204–214. doi: 10.1007/s12671-010-0029-y

Csikszentmihalyi, M., & Hunter, J. (2003). Happiness in everyday life: the uses of experience sampling. *Journal of Happiness Studies*, *4*, 185–199.

Cunningham, J., & Paradies, Y. C. (2012). Socio-demographic factors and psychological distress in Indigenous and non-Indigenous Australian adults aged 18–64 years: analysis of national survey data. *BMC Public Health*, *12*, 95. doi: 10.1186/1471-2458-12-95

Daaleman, T. P., & Dobbs, D. (2010). Religiosity, spirituality, and death attitudes in chronically ill older adults. *Research on Aging, 32*(2), 224–243.

Dallman, M. F., Pecoraro, N., Akana, S. F., La Fleur, S. E., Gomez, F., Houshyar, H., . . . Manalo, S. (2003). Chronic stress and obesity: a new view of 'comfort food'. *Proceedings of the National Academy of Sciences, 100*(20), 11696–11701. doi: 10.1073/pnas.1934666100

Darbonne, A., Uchino, B., & Ong, A. (2012). What mediates links between age and well-being? A test of social support and interpersonal conflict as potential interpersonal pathways. *Journal of Happiness Studies,* 1–13. doi: 10.1007/s10902-012-9363-1

Davidson, D. (1980). How is weakness of the will possible? *Essays on Actions and Events.* Oxford: Clarendon Press.

Department of Health (2010a). *Healthy foundations life-stage segmentation model toolkit.* London: Department of Health.

Department of Health (2010b). *Strategic review of health and social inequalities post-2010.* London: HMSO.

DeSalvo, K. B., Bloser, N., Reynolds, K., He, J., & Muntner, P. (2006). Mortality prediction with a single general self-rated health question. A meta-analysis. *Journal of General Internal Medicine, 21*(3), 267–275. doi: 10.1111/j.1525-1497.2005.00291.x

DeSalvo, K. B., & Muntner, P. (2011). Discordance between physician and patient self-rated health and all-cause mortality. *The Ochsner Journal, 11*(3), 232–240. doi: 10.1043/1524-5012-11.3.232

Dickerson, S. S., Gruenewald, T. L., & Kemeny, M. E. (2004). When the social self is threatened: shame, physiology, and health. *Journal of Personality, 72*(6), 1191–1216. doi: 10.1111/j.1467-6494.2004.00295.x

Diener, E., & Chan, M. Y. (2011). Happy people live longer: subjective well-being contributes to health and longevity. *Applied Psychology: Health and Well-Being, 3*(1), 1–43.

Diener, E., & Emmons, R. A. (1984). The independence of positive and negative affect. *J Pers Soc Psychol, 47*(5), 1105-1117.

Diener, E., Emmons, R. A., Larsen, R. J., & Griffin, S. (1985). The Satisfaction With Life Scale. *J Pers Assess, 49*(1), 71-75. doi: 10.1207/s15327752jpa4901_13

Diener, E., Ng, W., Harter, J., & Arora, R. (2010). Wealth and happiness across the world: material prosperity predicts life evaluation, whereas psychosocial prosperity predicts positive feeling. *Journal of Personality and Socal Psychology, 99*(1), 52–61. doi: 10.1037/a0018066

Diener, E., Suh, E. M., Lucas, R. E., & Smith, H. L. (1999). Subjective well-being: three decades of progress. *Psychological Bulletin, 125*(2), 276–302.

Dodd, D. K., Russell, B. L., & Jenkins, C. (1999). Smiling in school yearbook photos: gender differences from kindergarten to adulthood. *Psychological Record, 49*(4), 543–553.

Dolan, P., Layard, P. R. G., & Metcalfe, R. (2011). *Measuring well-being for public policy.* London: Office for National Statistics.

Douglas, I. (2012). Urban ecology and urban ecosystems: understanding the links to human health and well-being. *Current Opinion in Environmental Sustainability, 4*(4), 385–392. doi: http://dx.doi.org/10.1016/j.cosust.2012.07.005

Drentea, P., & Moren-Cross, J. L. (2005). Social capital and social support on the web: the case of an internet mother site. *Sociology Of Health & Illness, 7*, 920–943.

Dubé, L., LeBel, J. L., & Lu, J. (2005). Affect asymmetry and comfort food consumption. *Physiology & Behavior, 86*(4), 559–567. doi: 10.1016/j.physbeh.2005.08.023

Duchenne (de Boulogne), G.-B. (1876). *Mécanisme de la physionomie humaine ou analyse électro-physiologique de l'expression des passions. Texte: Deuxième partie (partie scientifique), Troisième partie (partie esthétique)*. Deuxième édition. Paris: Librairie J.-B. Bailliere et Fils.

Dyrdal, G. M., & Lucas, R. E. (2013). Reaction and adaptation to the birth of a child: a couple-level analysis. *Developmental Psychology, 49*(4), 749–761. doi: 10.1037/a0028335

Easterlin, R. A., McVey, L. A., Switek, M., Sawangfa, O., & Zweig, J. S. (2010). The happiness–income paradox revisited. *Proceedings of the National Academy of Sciences*.

Economic and Social Data Service (2012). *Guide to the 1970 British Cohort Study*. Retrieved 1 November 2012, from Universities of Essex and Manchester www.esds.ac.uk/longitudinal/access/bcs70/l33229.asp

Einstein, A. (1930). The world as I see it. *Forum and Century, 84*, 193–194.

Ekman, P. (2009). Darwin's contributions to our understanding of emotional expressions. *Philosophical Transactions of the Royal Society B: Biological Sciences, 364*(1535), 3449–3451.

Elliot, A. J., Sedikides, C., Murayama, K., Tanaka, A., Thrash, T. M., & Mapes, R. R. (2012). Cross-cultural generality and specificity in self-regulation: avoidance personal goals and multiple aspects of well-being in the United States and Japan. *Emotion, 12*(5), 1031–1040. doi: 10.1037/a0027456

Enck, P., Klosterhalfen, S., Weimer, K., Horing, B., & Zipfel, S. (2011). The placebo response in clinical trials: more questions than answers. *Philosophical Transactions of the Royal Society B: Biological Sciences, 366*(1572), 1889–1895.

Enkvist, A., Ekstrom, H., & Elmstahl, S. (2013). Associations between cognitive abilities and life satisfaction in the oldest-old. Results from the longitudinal population study Good Aging in Skane. *Journal of Clinical Interventions in Aging, 8*, 845–853. doi: 10.2147/cia.s45382

Entringer, S., Epel, E. S., Kumsta, R., Lin, J., Hellhammer, D. H., Blackburn, E. H., . . . Wadhwa, P. D. (2011). Stress exposure in intrauterine life is associated with shorter telomere length in young adulthood. *Proceedings of the National Academy of Sciences*.

Erikson, E., & Erikson, J. (1997). *The life-cycle completed* (Vol. 2). New York: W W Norton.

Eskine, K. J., Kacinik, N. A., & Prinz, J. J. (2011). A bad taste in the mouth. *Psychological Science, 22*(3), 295–299.

Etzioni, A. (2012). Communitarianism. In R. Chadwick (Ed.), *Encyclopedia of applied ethics* (2nd edn) (pp. 516–521). San Diego, CA: Academic Press.

Fagley, N. S. (2012). Appreciation uniquely predicts life satisfaction above demographics, the Big 5 personality factors, and gratitude. *Personality and Individual Differences, 53*(1), 59–63. doi: 10.1016/j.paid.2012.02.019

Farrington, D. (1995). The development of offending and antisocial behaviour from childhood: key findings from the Cambridge Study in Delinquent Behaviour. *Journal of Child Psychology and Psychiatry, 36,* 929–964.

Fernandez-Dols, J. M., & Ruiz-Belda, M. A. (1995). Are smiles a sign of happiness? Gold medal winners at the Olympic Games. *Journal of Personality and Social Psychology, 69*(6), 1113–1119.

Finkenauer, C., & Righetti, F. (2011). Understanding in close relationships: an interpersonal approach. *European Review of Social Psychology, 22*(1), 316–363. doi: 10.1080/10463283.2011.633384

Fletcher, S. K. (2004). Religion and life meaning: differentiating between religious beliefs and religious community in constructing life meaning. *Journal of Aging Studies, 18*(2), 171–185. doi: http://dx.doi.org/10.1016/j.jaging.2004.01.005

Foot, P. (1967). *The problem of abortion and the doctrine of the double effect in virtues and vices.* Oxford: Basil Blackwell, 1978. (Originally appeared in the *Oxford Review,* Number 5, 1967.)

Franco, M., Bilal, U., Orduñez, P., Benet, M., Morejón, A., Caballero, B., . . . Cooper, R. S. (2013). Population-wide weight loss and regain in relation to diabetes burden and cardiovascular mortality in Cuba 1980–2010: repeated cross sectional surveys and ecological comparison of secular trends. *British Medical Journal, 346.* doi: 10.1136/bmj.f1515

Frankl, V. E. (1963). *Man's search for meaning : an introduction to logotherapy.* New York: Washington Square Press.

Fredrickson, B. L. (2004). The broaden-and-build theory of positive emotions. *Philosophical Transactions of the Royal Society B: Biological Sciences, 359*(1449), 1367–1378. doi: 10.1098/rstb.2004.1512

Freud, S. (1913). *The interpretation of dreams.* New York: Macmillan.

Friedman, H. S., & Kern, M. L. (2013). Personality, well-being, and health. *Annual Review Of Psychology.* doi: 10.1146/annurev-psych-010213-115123

Fry, P. S., & Debats, D. L. (2011). Cognitive beliefs and future time perspectives: predictors of mortality and longevity. *Journal of Aging Research, 2011,* 367902. doi: 10.4061/2011/367902

Fujita, F., & Diener, E. (2005). Life satisfaction set point: stability and change. *Journal of Personality and Social Psychology, 88*(1), 158–164. doi: 10.1037/0022-3514.88.1.158

Fumagalli, M., Vergari, M., Pasqualetti, P., Marceglia, S., Mameli, F., Ferrucci, R., . . . Priori, A. (2010). Brain switches utilitarian behavior: does gender make the difference? *PLoS ONE, 5*(1), e8865. doi: 10.1371/journal.pone.0008865

Gale, C. R., Booth, T., Mõttus, R., Kuh, D., & Deary, I. J. (2013). Neuroticism and extraversion in youth predict mental wellbeing and life satisfaction 40 years later. *Journal of Research in Personality, 47*(6), 687–697. doi: http://dx.doi.org/10.1016/j.jrp.2013.06.005

Gall, T. L. (2006). Spirituality and coping with life stress among adult survivors of childhood sexual abuse. *Child Abuse & Neglect, 30*(7), 829–844. doi: http://dx.doi.org/10.1016/j.chiabu.2006.01.003

Gardner, J., & Oswald, A. J. (2007). Money and mental wellbeing: a longitudinal study of medium-sized lottery wins. *Journal of Health Economics, 26*(1), 49–60. doi: 10.1016/j.jhealeco.2006.08.004

Ghaemi, S. N. (2009). The rise and fall of the biopsychosocial model. *The British Journal of Psychiatry, 195*(1), 3–4.

Giddens, A. (1991). *Modernity and self-identity*. Cambridge, UK: Polity Press.

Gilbert, P., & Allan, S. (1998). The role of defeat and entrapment (arrested flight) in depression: an exploration of an evolutionary view. *Psychological Medicine, 28*(3), 585–598.

Gilbert, P., Allan, S., Brough, S., Melley, S., & Miles, J. N. V. (2002). Relationship of anhedonia and anxiety to social rank, defeat and entrapment. *Journal of Affective Disorders, 71*(1–3), 141–151. doi: 10.1016/s0165-0327(01)00392-5

Gleichgerrcht, E., & Young, L. (2013). Low levels of empathic concern predict utilitarian moral judgment. *PLoS ONE, 8*(4), e60418. doi: 10.1371/journal.pone.0060418

Goffman, E. (1963). *Stigma; notes on the management of spoiled identity*. Englewood Cliffs, NJ: Prentice-Hall.

Goffman, E. (1969). On face work. In *Where the action is* (pp. 1–36). London: Allen Lane.

Gray, H. M., Ishii, K., & Ambady, N. (2011). Misery loves company: when sadness increases the desire for social connectedness. *Personality & Social Psychology Bulletin, 37*(11), 1438–1448. doi: 10.1177/0146167211420167

Grayling, A. (2007). *The choice of Hercules*. London: Weidenfeld and Nicolson.

Green, J. G., McLaughlin, K. A., Berglund, P. A., Gruber, M. J., Sampson, N. A., Zaslavsky, A. M., & Kessler, R. C. (2010). Childhood adversities and adult psychiatric disorders in the national comorbidity survey replication I: associations with first onset of *DSM-IV* disorders. *Archives Of General Psychiatry, 67*(2), 113–123. doi: 10.1001/archgenpsychiatry.2009.186

Grosbras, M.-H., Tan, H., & Pollick, F. (2012). Dance and emotion in posterior parietal cortex: a low-frequency rTMS study. *Brain Stimulation, 5*(2), 130–136. doi: 10.1016/j.brs.2012.03.013

Grossmann, T., Johnson, M. H., Vaish, A., Hughes, D. A., Quinque, D., Stoneking, M., & Friederici, A. D. (2011). Genetic and neural dissociation of individual responses to emotional expressions in human infants. *Developmental Cognitive Neuroscience, 1*(1), 57–66.

Gruber, J., Johnson, S. L., Oveis, C., & Keltner, D. (2008). Risk for mania and positive emotional responding: too much of a good thing? *Emotion, 8*(1), 23–33.

Haase, C. M., Poulin, M. J., & Heckhausen, J. (2012). Happiness as a motivator: positive affect predicts primary control striving for career and rducational goals. *Personality & Social Psychology Bulletin*. doi: 10.1177/0146167212444906

Hare, E. (2001). Weakness of will. In L. Becker & C. Becker (Eds), *The Encyclopedia of Ethics* (2nd edn, pp. 1789–1792). New York: Routledge.

Hawker, C. L. (2012). Physical activity and mental well-being in student nurses. *Nurse Education Today, 32*(3), 325–331. doi: 10.1016/j.nedt.2011.07.013

Hawkes, N. (2012). NHS spending should focus on mental rather than physical health to promote wellbeing. *British Medical Journal, 345*. doi: 10.1136/bmj.e7914

Health and Social Care Information Centre (2011). *Attitudes to mental illness*. London: Health and Social Care Information Centre.

Hecht, D. (2010). Depression and the hyperactive right-hemisphere. *Neuroscience Research*, *68*(2), 77–87. doi: 10.1016/j.neures.2010.06.013

Heidinger, B. J., Blount, J. D., Boner, W., Griffiths, K., Metcalfe, N. B., & Monaghan, P. (2012). Telomere length in early life predicts lifespan. *Proceedings of the National Academy of Sciences*.

Helliwell, J. F., & Barrington-Leigh, C. (2010). *How much is social capital worth?* Retrieved from http://ssrn.com/abstract=1612617

Helliwell, J. F., Layard, R., & Sachs, J. (Eds) (2012). *World happiness report*. New York: The Earth Institute, Columbia University.

Hepper, E. G., Ritchie, T. D., Sedikides, C., & Wildschut, T. (2012). Odyssey's end: lay conceptions of nostalgia reflect its original Homeric meaning. *Emotion*, *12*(1), 102–119. doi: 10.1037/a0025167

Heritage, Z. (2009). Inequalities, social ties and health in France. *Public Health*, *123*(1), e29–e34.

Hobbs, N., Dixon, D., Johnston, M., & Howie, K. (2013). Can the theory of planned behaviour predict the physical activity behaviour of individuals? *Psychology & Health*, *28*(3), 234–249. doi: 10.1080/08870446.2012.716838

Hofmann, W., Luhmann, M., Fisher, R. R., Vohs, K. D., & Baumeister, R. F. (2013). Yes, but are they happy? Effects of trait self-control on affective well-being and life satisfaction. *Journal Of Personality*. doi: 10.1111/jopy.12050

Hsu, H.-C. (2010). Trajectory of life satisfaction and its relationship with subjective economic status and successful aging. *Social Indicators Research*, *99*(3), 455–468. doi: 10.1007/s11205-010-9593-8

Hsu, L. M., Chung, J., & Langer, E. J. (2010). The influence of age-related cues on health and longevity. *Perspectives on Psychological Science*, *5*(6), 632–648.

Huang, J., & Bargh, J. (to be published). The selfish goal: autonomously operating motivational structures as the proximate cause of human judgment and behavior. *Behavioral and Brain Science*.

Huber, M., Knottnerus, J. A., Green, L., van der Horst, H., Jadad, A. R., Kromhout, D., . . . Smid, H. (2011). How should we define health? *British Medical Journal*, *343*. doi: 10.1136/bmj.d4163

Huffmeijer, R., Alink, L. R., Tops, M., Grewen, K. M., Light, K. C., Bakermans-Kranenburg, M. J., & van Ijzendoorn, M. H. (2012). The impact of oxytocin administration and maternal love withdrawal on event-related potential (ERP) responses to emotional faces with performance feedback. *Hormones and Behavior*. doi: 10.1016/j.yhbeh.2012.11.008

Huppert, F., & So, T. C. (2013). Flourishing across Europe: application of a new conceptual framework for defining well-being. *Social Indicators Research*, *110*(3), 837-861. doi: 10.1007/s11205-011-9966-7

Hutcherson, C. A., Seppala, E. M., & Gross, J. J. (2008). Loving-kindness meditation increases social connectedness. *Emotion*, *8*(5), 720–724.

Hutnik, N., Smith, P., & Koch, T. (2012). What does it feel like to be 100? Socio-emotional aspects of well-being in the stories of 16 centenarians living in the United Kingdom. *Aging & Mental Health*, *16*(7), 811–818. doi: 10.1080/13607863.2012.684663

Ironson, G., & Kremer, H. (2009). Spiritual transformation, psychological well-being, health, and survival in people with HIV. *International Journal of Psychiatry in Medicine, 39*(3), 263–281.

Janis, I. L. (1983). Stress inoculation in health care: theory and research. In D. Meichenbaum & M. Jaremko (Eds), *Stress reduction and prevention* (pp. 67–100). New York: Plenum.

Janoff-Bulman, R. (1992). *Shattered assumptions: towards a new psychology of trauma*. New York: Free Press; Toronto: Maxwell Macmillan Canada; New York: Maxwell Macmillan International.

Jefferson, T. (1903). *Memorial edition* (Vol. 16). Washington, DC: Lipscomb and Bergh.

Judge, T., Ilies, R., & Dimotakis, N. (2010). Are health and happiness the product of wisdom? The relationship of general mental ability to educational and occupational attainment, health, and well-being. *Journal of Applied Psychology, 95*(3), 454–468. doi: 10.1037/a0019084

Jung, C. G. (1923). *Psychological types: or, The psychology of individuation*. London: Kegan Paul.

Kagan, J., & Snidman, N. (1999). Early childhood predictors of adult anxiety disorders. *Biological Psychiatry, 46*(11), 1536–1541.

Kahane, G. U. Y., & Shackel, N. (2010). Methodological issues in the neuroscience of moral judgement. *Mind & Language, 25*(5), 561–582. doi: 10.1111/j.1468-0017.2010.01401.x

Kahneman, D. (2006). Determinants of health economic decisions in actual practice: the role of behavioral economics. Summary of the presentation given by Professor Daniel Kahneman at the ISPOR 10th Annual International Meeting First Plenary Session, May 16, 2005, Washington, DC, USA. *Value Health, 9*(2), 65–67. doi: 10.1111/j.1524-4733.2006.00084.x

Kahneman, D., Krueger, A. B., Schkade, D. A., Schwarz, N., & Stone, A. A. (2004). A survey method for characterizing daily life experience: the day reconstruction method. *Science, 306*(5702), 1776–1780. doi: 10.1126/science.1103572

Kahneman, D., & Tversky, A. (1979). Prospect theory: an analysis of decision under risk. *Econometrica, 47*(2), 263–291.

Kaptchuk, T. J., Friedlander, E., Kelley, J. M., Sanchez, M. N., Kokkotou, E., Singer, J. P., . . . Lembo, A. J. (2010). Placebos without deception: a randomized controlled trial in Irritable Bowel Syndrome. *PLoS ONE, 5*(12), e15591. doi: 10.1371/journal.pone.0015591

Kark, J. D., Shemi, G., Friedlander, Y., Martin, O., Manor, O., & Blondheim, S. H. (1996). Does religious observance promote health? mortality in secular vs religious kibbutzim in Israel. *Am J Public Health, 86*(3), 341–346.

Kashdan, T. B., Weeks, J. W., & Savostyanova, A. A. (2011). Whether, how, and when social anxiety shapes positive experiences and events: a self-regulatory framework and treatment implications. *Clinical Psychology Review, 31*(5), 786–799. doi: 10.1016/j.cpr.2011.03.012

Kato, K., Zweig, R., Barzilai, N., & Atzmon, G. (2012). Positive attitude towards life and emotional expression as personality phenotypes for centenarians. *Aging* (Albany NY), *4*(5), 359–367.

Keeley, B. (2007). *Human capital*. Paris: OECD.

Kendler, K. S., & Halberstadt, L. J. (2012). The road not taken: life experiences in monozygotic twin pairs discordant for major depression. *Molecular Psychiatry*. doi: 10.1038/mp.2012.55

Keng, S. L., Smoski, M. J., & Robins, C. J. (2011). Effects of mindfulness on psychological health: a review of empirical studies. *Clinical Psychology Review, 31*(6), 1041–1056. doi: 10.1016/j.cpr.2011.04.006

Keyes, C., Myers, J., & Kendler, K. (2010). The structure of the genetic and environmental influences on mental well-being. *American Journal of Public Health, 100*(12), 2379–2384. doi: 10.2105/AJPH.2010.193615

Keyes, C. L. M. (2005). Mental illness and/or mental health? Investigating axioms of the complete state model of health [report]. *Journal of Consulting & Clinical Psychology, 73*(3), 539–548.

Khor, A. S., Gray, K. M., Reid, S. C., & Melvin, G. A. (2014). Feasibility and validity of ecological momentary assessment in adolescents with high-functioning autism and Asperger's disorder. *Journal of Adolescence, 37*(1), 37–46. doi: http://dx.doi.org/10.1016/j.adolescence.2013.10.005

Kierkegaard, S. (1988 (1844)). *Kierkegaard's writings, XI: Stages on life's way.* Princeton: Princeton University Press.

Kinnier, R. T., Kernes, J. L., Tribbensee, N. E., & Van Puymbroeck, C. M. (2003). What eminent people have said about the meaning of life. *Journal of Humanistic Psychology, 43*(1), 105–118.

Kiser, D., Steemers, B., Branchi, I., & Homberg, J. R. (2012). The reciprocal interaction between serotonin and social behaviour. *Neuroscience & Biobehavioral Reviews, 36*(2), 786–798. doi: 10.1016/j.neubiorev.2011.12.009

Knoch, D., Nitsche, M. A., Fischbacher, U., Eisenegger, C., Pascual-Leone, A., & Fehr, E. (2008). Studying the neurobiology of social interaction with transcranial direct current stimulation – the example of punishing unfairness. *Cerebral Cortex, 18*(9), 1987–1990.

Koivumaa-Honkanen, H., Kaprio, J., Honkanen, R. J., Viinamaki, H., & Koskenvuo, M. (2005). The stability of life satisfaction in a 15-year follow-up of adult Finns healthy at baseline. *BMC Psychiatry, 5,* 4. doi: 10.1186/1471-244x-5-4

Kok, B. E., Coffey, K. A., Cohn, M. A., Catalino, L. I., Vacharkulksemsuk, T., Algoe, S. B., . . . Fredrickson, B. L. (2013). How positive emotions build physical health: perceived positive social connections account for the upward spiral between positive emotions and vagal tone. *Psychological Science, 24*(7), 1123–1132. doi: 10.1177/0956797612470827

Kokko, K., Tolvanen, A., & Pulkkinen, L. (2013). Associations between personality traits and psychological well-being across time in middle adulthood. *Journal of Research in Personality, 47*(6), 748–756. doi: http://dx.doi.org/10.1016/j.jrp.2013.07.002

Konopack, J. F., & McAuley, E. (2012). Efficacy-mediated effects of spirituality and physical activity on quality of life: a path analysis. *Health and Quality of Life Outcomes, 10,* 57. doi: 10.1186/1477-7525-10-57

Koole, S. L. (2008). The psychology of emotion regulation: an integrative review. *Cognition & Emotion, 23*(1), 4–41. doi: 10.1080/02699930802619031

Kron, A., Schul, Y., Cohen, A., & Hassin, R. R. (2010). Feelings don't come easy: studies on the effortful nature of feelings. *Journal of Experimental Psychology: General, 139*(3), 520–534. doi: 10.1037/a0020008

LaFrance, M., Hecht, M. A., & Paluck, E. L. (2003). The contingent smile: a meta-analysis of sex differences in smiling. *Psychological Bulletin, 129*(2), 305–334.

Larsen, B. A., Darby, R. S., Harris, C. R., Nelkin, D. K., Milam, P.-E., & Christenfeld, N. J. S. (2012). The immediate and delayed cardiovascular benefits of forgiving. *Psychosomatic Medicine, 74*(7), 745–750. doi: 10.1097/PSY.0b013e31825fe96c

Lawlor, D. A., & Hopker, S. W. (2001). The effectiveness of exercise as an intervention in the management of depression: systematic review and meta-regression analysis of randomised controlled trials. *British Medical Journal, 322*(7289), 763. doi: 10.1136/bmj.322.7289.763

Layard, P. R. G. (2011). *Happiness: lessons from a new science* (2nd edn). London: Penguin Press.

Layard, R., Clark, A. E., & Senik, C. (2012). The causes of happiness and misery. In J. F. Helliwell, R. Layard & J. Sachs (Eds), *The world happiness report* (pp. 58–89). New York: The Earth Institute, Columbia University.

Lazarus, R. S., & Folkman, S. (1984). *Stress, appraisal, and coping.* New York: Springer Pub. Co.

Leach, C. W., & Spears, R. (2008). 'A vengefulness of the impotent': the pain of in-group inferiority and schadenfreude toward successful out-groups. *Journal of Personality and Social Psychology, 95*(6), 1383–1396. doi: 10.1037/a0012629

Leach, L. S., Butterworth, P., Olesen, S. C., & Mackinnon, A. (2012). Relationship quality and levels of depression and anxiety in a large population-based survey. *Social Psychiatry and Psychiatric Epidemiology.* doi: 10.1007/s00127-012-0559-9

Lee, R. M., Dean, B. L., & Jung, K.-R. (2008). Social connectedness, extraversion, and subjective well-being: testing a mediation model. *Personality and Individual Differences, 45*(5), 414–419. doi: http://dx.doi.org/10.1016/j.paid.2008.05.017

Leith, K. P., & Baumeister, R. F. (1996). Why do bad moods increase self-defeating behavior? Emotion, risk tasking, and self-regulation. *Journal of Personality and Social Psychology, 71*(6), 1250–1267.

Leserman, J., Petitto, J. M., Golden, R. N., Gaynes, B. N., Gu, H., Perkins, D. O., . . . Evans, D. L. (2000). Impact of stressful life events, depression, social support, coping, and cortisol on progression to AIDS. *The American Journal of Psychiatry, 157*(8), 1221–1228.

Lesh, T. V. (1970a). The relationship between Zen meditation and the development of accurate empathy. *Dissertation Abstracts International,* (11-A), 4778–4779.

Lesh, T. V. (1970b). Zen meditation and the development of empathy in counselors. *Journal of Humanistic Psychology,* (1), 39–74.

Lewis, C. A., & Cruise, S. M. (2006). Religion and happiness: consensus, contradictions, comments and concerns. *Mental Health, Religion & Culture, 9*(3), 213–225. doi: 10.1080/13694670600615276

Light, S. N., Coan, J. A., Frye, C., Goldsmith, H. H., & Davidson, R. J. (2009). Dynamic variation in pleasure in children predicts nonlinear change in lateral frontal brain electrical activity. *Developmental Psychology, 45*(2), 525–533. doi: 10.1037/a0014576

Light, S. N., Coan, J. A., Zahn-Waxler, C., Frye, C., Goldsmith, H. H., & Davidson, R. J. (2009). Empathy is associated with dynamic change in prefrontal brain electrical activity during positive emotion in children. *Child Development, 80*(4), 1210–1231. doi: 10.1111/j.1467-8624.2009.01326.x

Lo, C., Zimmermann, C., Gagliese, L., Li, M., & Rodin, G. (2011). Sources of spiritual well-being in advanced cancer. *BMJ Supportive & Palliative Care, 1*(2), 149–153.

Lucas, R. E. (2007). Long-term disability is associated with lasting changes in subjective well-being: evidence from two nationally representative longitudinal studies. *Journal of Personality and Social Psychology, 92*(4), 717–730. doi: 10.1037/0022-3514.92.4.717

Lucas, R. E., Clark, A. E., Georgellis, Y., & Diener, E. (2003). Reexamining adaptation and the set point model of happiness: reactions to changes in marital status. *Journal of Personality and Social Psychology, 84*(3), 527–539. doi: 10.1037/0022-3514.84.3.527

Luhmann, M., Hawkley, L. C., Eid, M., & Cacioppo, J. T. (2012). Time frames and the distinction between affective and cognitive well-being. *Journal of Research in Personality, 46*(4), 431–441. doi: 10.1016/j.jrp.2012.04.004

Ly, H. (2009). Genetic and environmental factors influencing human diseases with telomere dysfunction. *International Journal of Clinical and Experimental Medicine, 2*(2), 114–130.

Lykken, D., & Tellegen, A. (1996). Happiness is a stochastic phenomenon. *Psychological Science, 7*(3), 186–189.

Maddi, S. R., & Kobasa, S. C. (1984). *The hardy executive: health under stress.* Homewood, IL: Dow Jones-Irwin.

Madigan, S., Atkinson, L., Laurin, K., & Benoit, D. (2013). Attachment and internalizing behavior in early childhood: a meta-analysis. *Developmental Psychology, 49*(4), 672–689. doi: 10.1037/a0028793

Mainguy, B., Valenti Pickren, M., & Mehl-Madrona, L. (2013). Relationships between level of spiritual transformation and medical outcome. *Advances in Mind–Body Medicine, 27*(1), 4–11.

Mar, R. A., Mason, M. F., & Litvack, A. (2012). How daydreaming relates to life satisfaction, loneliness, and social support: the importance of gender and daydream content. *Consciousness and Cognition, 21*(1), 401–407. doi: 10.1016/j.concog.2011.08.001

Marchant, E. C. (1923). *Xenophon in seven volumes.* London: Heinemann Ltd.

Marmot, M. (2004). *The status syndrome.* London: Bloomsbury.

Maslow, A. (1968). *Toward a psychology of being.* New York: Van Nostrand Co.

Matthews, C. E., Jurj, A. L., Shu, X.-o., Li, H.-L., Yang, G., Li, Q., . . . Zheng, W. (2007). Influence of exercise, walking, cycling, and overall nonexercise physical activity on mortality in Chinese women. *American Journal of Epidemiology, 165*(12), 1343–1350.

Mauss, I. B., Shallcross, A. J., Troy, A. S., John, O. P., Ferrer, E., Wilhelm, F. H., & Gross, J. J. (2011). Don't hide your happiness! Positive emotion dissociation, social connectedness, and psychological functioning. *Journal of Personality and Social Psychology, 100*(4), 738–748. doi: 10.1037/a0022410

May, R. (1950). *The meaning of anxiety.* New York: W. W. Norton.

Mazzucchelli, T. G., Kane, R. T., & Rees, C. S. (2010). Behavioral activation interventions for well-being: a meta-analysis. *The Journal of Positive Psychology, 5*(2), 105–121. doi: 10.1080/17439760903569154

Meeks, T. W. M., & Jeste, D. V. M. (2009). Neurobiology of wisdom: a literature overview. *Archives Of General Psychiatry, 66*(4), 355.

Mele, A. R. (2000). Self-deception and emotion. *Consciousness & Emotion, 1*(1), 115–137. doi: 10.1075/ce.1.1.07mel

Michie, S., van Stralen, M. M., & West, R. (2011). The behaviour change wheel: a new method for characterising and designing behaviour change interventions. *Implementation Science*, (6), 42. doi: 10.1186/1748-5908-6-42

Michie, S., Richardson, M., Johnston, M., Abraham, C., Francis, J., Hardeman, W., . . . Wood, C. E. (2013). The behavior change technique taxonomy (v1) of 93 hierarchically clustered techniques: building an international consensus for the reporting of behavior change interventions. *Annals of behavioral medicine: a publication of the Society of Behavioral Medicine*, 46(1), 81–95. doi: 10.1007/s12160-013-9486-6

Mileva-Seitz, V., Steiner, M., Atkinson, L., Meaney, M. J., Levitan, R., Kennedy, J. L., . . . Fleming, A. S. (2013). Interaction between oxytocin genotypes and early experience predicts quality of mothering and postpartum mood. *PLoS ONE*, 8(4), e61443. doi: 10.1371/journal.pone.0061443

Mill, J. S. (1867). *Utilitarianism* (3rd edn). London: Longmans, Green, Reader & Dyer.

Mill, J. S. (1909). *Autobiography*. New York: P F Collier and Son.

Miller, G. A. (2010). Mistreating psychology in the decades of the brain. *Perspectives on Psychological Science*, 5(6), 716–743.

Moberg, D., & Taves, M. (1965). Church participation and adjustment in old age. In A. Rose & W. Peterson (Eds), *Older people and their social world* (pp. 113–124). Philadelphia: F A Davis.

Moffitt, T. E., Arseneault, L., Belsky, D., Dickson, N., Hancox, R. J., Harrington, H., . . . Caspi, A. (2011). A gradient of childhood self-control predicts health, wealth, and public safety. *Proceedings of the National Academy of Sciences*, 108(7), 2693–2698.

Moll, J., & de Oliveira-Souza, R. (2007). Moral judgments, emotions and the utilitarian brain. *Trends in Cognitive Sciences*, 11(8), 319–321.

Mukuria, C., & Brazier, J. (2013). Valuing the EQ-5D and the SF-6D health states using subjective well-being: a secondary analysis of patient data. *Social Science & Medicine*, 77(0), 97–105. doi: http://dx.doi.org/10.1016/j.socscimed.2012.11.012

Murphy, J. M., Olivier, D. C., Monson, R. R., Sobol, A. M., Federman, E. B., & Leighton, A. H. (1991). Depression and anxiety in relation to social status: a prospective epidemiologic study. *Archives Of General Psychiatry*, 48(3), 223–229. doi: 10.1001/archpsyc.1991.01810270035004

Murphy, S. A., & Johnson, L. C. (2003). Finding meaning in a child's violent death: a five-year prospective analysis of parents' personal narratives and empirical data. *Death Studies*, 27(5), 381–404.

Myers, D. G. (2000). The funds, friends, and faith of happy people. *American Psychologist*, 55(1), 56–67. doi: 10.1037/0003-066x.55.1.56

Mykletun, A., Bjerkeset, O., Øverland, S., Prince, M., Dewey, M., & Stewart, R. (2009). Levels of anxiety and depression as predictors of mortality: the HUNT study. *The British Journal of Psychiatry*, 195(2), 118–125.

Nagashima, A., & Touhara, K. (2010). Enzymatic conversion of odorants in nasal mucus affects olfactory glomerular activation patterns and odor perception. *The Journal of Neuroscience*, 30(48), 16391–16398. doi: 10.1523/jneurosci.2527-10.2010

Nakamura, K.-I., Takubo, K., Izumiyama-Shimomura, N., Sawabe, M., Arai, T., Kishimoto, H., . . . Ishikawa, N. (2007). Telomeric DNA length in cerebral gray and white matter is associated with longevity in individuals aged 70 years or older. *Experimental Gerontology*, 42(10), 944–950. doi: 10.1016/j.exger.2007.05.003

Newman, J. A. (1994). Affective empathy training with senior citizens using Zazen (zen) meditation. *Dissertation Abstracts International Section A: Humanities and Social Sciences, 55*(5-A), 1193.

Neyt, M., & Albrecht, J. (2006). The long-term evolution of quality of life for disease-free breast cancer survivors: a comparative study in Belgium. *Journal of Psychosocial Oncology, 24*(3), 89–123. doi: 10.1300/J077v24n03_05

Ng, K. H., Agius, M., & Zaman, R. (2011). P01-557 – Effect of the worldwide crises on mental health. *European Psychiatry, 26*, Supplement 1, 561. doi: 10.1016/s0924-9338(11)72268-4

Ni Mhaolain, A. M., Gallagher, D., O'Connell, H., Chin, A. V., Bruce, I., Hamilton, F., . . . Lawlor, B. A. (2012). Subjective well-being amongst community-dwelling elders: what determines satisfaction with life? Findings from the Dublin Healthy Aging Study. *International psychogeriatrics/IPA, 24*(2), 316–323. doi: 10.1017/S1041610211001360

Niemi, A.-K., Hervonen, A., Hurme, M., Karhunen, P., Jylhä, M., & Majamaa, K. (2003). Mitochondrial DNA polymorphisms associated with longevity in a Finnish population. *Human Genetics, 112*(1), 29–33. doi: 10.1007/s00439-002-0843-y

Nietzsche, F. (1882/2001). *The gay science*. Cambridge: Cambridge University Press.

Nisbett, R. E., Caputo, C., Legant, P., & Maracek, J. (1973). Behaviour as seen by the actor and as seen by the observer. *Journal of Personality and Social Psychology, 27,* 154–164.

Nozick, R. (1974). *Anarchy, state, and utopia*. New York: Basic Books.

O'Reilly, D., & Rosato, M. (2010). Dissonances in self-reported health and mortality across denominational groups in Northern Ireland. *Social Science & Medicine, 71*(5), 1011–1017. doi: 10.1016/j.socscimed.2010.05.042

Obrien, L. V., Berry, H. L., & Hogan, A. (2012). The structure of psychological life satisfaction: insights from farmers and a general community sample in Australia. *BMC Public Health, 12*(1), 976. doi: 10.1186/1471-2458-12-976

Oerlemans, W. G., Bakker, A. B., & Veenhoven, R. (2011). Finding the key to happy aging: a day reconstruction study of happiness. *The Journals of Gerontology. Series B, Psychological Sciences and Social Sciences, 66*(6), 665–674. doi: 10.1093/geronb/gbr040

Oksuzyan, A., Maier, H., McGue, M., Vaupel, J. W., & Christensen, K. (2010). Sex differences in the level and rate of change of physical function and grip strength in the Danish 1905-Cohort Study. *Journal of Aging and Health, 22*(5), 589–610.

Oreopoulos, P., & Salvanes, K. G. (2011). Priceless: the nonpecuniary benefits of schooling. *Journal of Economic Perspectives, 25*(1), 159–184.

Ost, L. G. (1996). One-session group treatment of spider phobia. *Behaviour Research And Therapy, 34*(9), 707–715.

Peirce, C. (1958). *Selected writings*. New York: Dover.

Pelham, B. W., Mirenberg, M. C., & Jones, J. T. (2002). Why Susie sells seashells by the seashore: implicit egotism and major life decisions. *Journal of Personality and Social Psychology, 82*(4), 469–487.

Penrose, R. (1999). *The Emperor's new mind* (Paperback ed). Oxford: Oxford University Press.

Perry, J. C., & Bond, M. (2012). Change in defense mechanisms during long-term dynamic psychotherapy and five-year outcome. *The American Journal of Psychiatry*. doi: 10.1176/appi.ajp.2012.11091403

Peterson, C. F., & Seligman, M. E. P. (2004). *Character strengths and virtues: a handbook and classification.* Washington, D.C.: American Psychological Association; Oxford: Oxford University Press.

Peterson, F., & Jung, C. G. (1907). Psycho-physical investigations with the galvanometer and pneumograph in normal and insane individuals. *Brain, 30*(2), 153–218.

Pevalin, D. J., & Rose, D. (2003). *Social capital for health: investigating the links between social capital and health using the British Household Panel Survey.* NHS Health Development Agency.

Pilkington, P. D., Windsor, T. D., & Crisp, D. A. (2012). Volunteering and subjective well-being in midlife and older adults: the role of supportive social networks. *The Journals of Gerontology. Series B, Psychological Sciences and Social Sciences, 67*(2), 249–260. doi: 10.1093/geronb/gbr154

Pinquart, M. (2001). Correlates of subjective health in older adults: a meta-analysis. *Psychology and Aging, 16*(3), 414–426. doi: 10.1037/0882-7974.16.3.414

Pirmohamed, M. (2011). Pharmacogenetics: past, present and future. *Drug Discovery Today, 16*(19–20), 852–861. doi: 10.1016/j.drudis.2011.08.006

Pressman, S. D., Gallagher, M. W., & Lopez, S. J. (2013). Is the emotion–health connection a 'first-world problem'? *Psychological Science, 24*(4), 544–549. doi: 10.1177/0956797612457382

Price, N. L., Gomes, A. P., Ling, A. J. Y., Duarte, F. V., Martin-Montalvo, A., North, B. J., . . . Sinclair, D. A. (2012). SIRT1 is required for AMPK activation and the beneficial effects of resveratrol on mitochondrial function. *Cell Metabolism, 15*(5), 675–690.

Price, R. H., Choi, J. N., & Vinokur, A. D. (2002). Links in the chain of adversity following job loss: how financial strain and loss of personal control lead to depression, impaired functioning, and poor health. *Journal of Occupational Health Psychology, 7*(4), 302–312.

Prilleltensky, I. (2012). Wellness as fairness. *American Journal of Community Psychology, 49*(1–2), 1–21. doi: 10.1007/s10464-011-9448-8

Proulx, C. M., & Snyder-Rivas, L. A. (2013). The longitudinal associations between marital happiness, problems, and self-rated health. *Journal of Family Psychology, 27*(2), 194–202. doi: 10.1037/a0031877

Putnam, R. D. (2000). *Bowling alone: the collapse and revival of American community.* New York; London: Simon & Schuster.

Rantanen, T., Masaki, K., He, Q., Ross, G., Willcox, B., & White, L. (2012). Midlife muscle strength and human longevity up to age 100 years: a 44-year prospective study among a decedent cohort. *AGE, 34*(3), 563–570. doi: 10.1007/s11357-011-9256-y

Recio, G., Sommer, W., & Schacht, A. (2011). Electrophysiological correlates of perceiving and evaluating static and dynamic facial emotional expressions. *Brain Research, 1376*(0), 66–75. doi: 10.1016/j.brainres.2010.12.041

Reynolds, S. L., Haley, W. E., & Kozlenko, N. (2008). The impact of depressive symptoms and chronic diseases on active life expectancy in older Americans. *The American Journal of Geriatric Psychiatry, 16*(5), 425–432. doi: http://dx.doi.org/10.1097/JGP.0b013e31816ff32e

Riedl, M. (2012). The containment of Dionysos: religion and politics in the Bacchanalia Affair of 186 BCE. *International Political Anthropology, 5*(2), 113–133.

Rief, W., Nestoriuc, Y., Weiss, S., Welzel, E., Barsky, A. J., & Hofmann, S. G. (2009). Meta-analysis of the placebo response in antidepressant trials. *Journal of Affective Disorders*, *118*(1–3), 1–8. doi: 10.1016/j.jad.2009.01.029

Robinson, O. J., Charney, D. R., Overstreet, C., Vytal, K., & Grillon, C. (2012). The adaptive threat bias in anxiety: amygdala, dorsomedial prefrontal cortex coupling and aversive amplification. *Neuroimage*, *60*(1), 523–529. doi: 10.1016/j.neuroimage.2011.11.096

Rogers, S. (2012). Bobby Kennedy on GDP: 'measures everything except that which is worthwhile'. *The Guardian*. Retrieved from www.theguardian.com/news/datablog/2012/may/24/robert-kennedy-gdp

Rowsell, H., & Coplan, R. (2012). Exploring links between shyness, romantic relationship quality, and well-being. *Canadian Journal of Behavioural Science/Revue canadienne des sciences du comportement*, *45*(4), 287–295. doi: 10.1037/a0029853

Ruis, M. A., te Brake, J. H., Buwalda, B., de Boer, S. F., Meerlo, P., Korte, S. M., . . . Koolhaas, J. M. (1999). Housing familiar male wildtype rats together reduces the long-term adverse behavioural and physiological effects of social defeat. *Psychoneuroendocrinology*, *24*(3), 285–300.

Russ, T. C., Stamatakis, E., Hamer, M., Starr, J. M., Kivimäki, M., & Batty, G. D. (2012). Association between psychological distress and mortality: individual participant pooled analysis of 10 prospective cohort studies. *British Medical Journal*, *345*. doi: 10.1136/bmj.e4933

Russell, B. (1968 (1930)). *The conquest of happiness*. New York: Bantam.

Ryff, C., Burton, H., & Love, D. (2004). Positive health: connecting well-being with biology. *Philosophical Transactions of the Royal Society of London. Series B: Biological Sciences*, *359*(1449), 1383–1394.

Ryle, G. (2009). *The concept of mind* (60th anniversary edn). Abingdon: Routledge.

Sartre, J. P. (1971). *Sketch for a theory of the emotions*. London: Methuen and Co.

Sato, W., Kochiyama, T., Uono, S., & Yoshikawa, S. (2010). Amygdala integrates emotional expression and gaze direction in response to dynamic facial expressions. *Neuroimage*, *50*(4), 1658–1665. doi: 10.1016/j.neuroimage.2010.01.049

Saunders, T., Driskell, J. E., Johnston, J. H., & Salas, E. (1996). The effect of stress inoculation training on anxiety and performance. *Journal of Occupational Health Psychology*, *1*(2), 170–186.

Scheid, C., Schmidt, J., & Noë, R. (2008). Distinct patterns of food offering and co-feeding in rooks. *Animal Behaviour*, *76*(5), 1701–1707. doi: 10.1016/j.anbehav.2008.07.023

Scheler, M. (1994). *Ressentiment* (new edn). Milwaukee: Marquette University Press.

Schimmack, U., Oishi, S., Furr, R. M., & Funder, D. C. (2004). Personality and life satisfaction: A Facet-Level Analysis. *Personality and Social Psychology Bulletin*, *30*(8), 1062-1075. doi: 10.1177/0146167204264292

Schneiderman, I., Zagoory-Sharon, O., Leckman, J. F., & Feldman, R. (2012). Oxytocin during the initial stages of romantic attachment: relations to couples' interactive reciprocity. *Psychoneuroendocrinology*, *37*(8), 1277–1285. doi: 10.1016/j.psyneuen.2011.12.021

Schützwohl, A., & Reisenzein, R. (2012). Facial expressions in response to a highly surprising event exceeding the field of vision: a test of Darwin's theory of surprise. *Evolution and Human Behavior*, *33*(6), 657–664. doi: http://dx.doi.org/10.1016/j.evolhumbehav.2012.04.003

Seaford, C. (2011). Policy: time to legislate for the good life. *Nature*, *477*(7366), 532–533. doi: 10.1038/477532a

Seawell, A. H., Toussaint, L. L., & Cheadle, A. C. (2013). Prospective associations between unforgiveness and physical health and positive mediating mechanisms in a nationally representative sample of older adults. *Psychology & Health*. doi: 10.1080/08870446.2013.856434

Seery, M. D., Holman, E. A., & Silver, R. C. (2010). Whatever does not kill us: cumulative lifetime adversity, vulnerability, and resilience. *Journal of Personality and Social Psychology*. doi: 10.1037/a0021344

Seeyave, D. M. M., Coleman, S. M. P. H., Appugliese, D. M. P. H., Corwyn, R. F. P., Bradley, R. H. P., Davidson, N. S. P., . . . Lumeng, J. C. M. (2009). Ability to delay gratification at age 4 years and risk of overweight at age 11 years. *Archives of Pediatrics & Adolescent Medicine*, *163*(4), 303.

Selezneva, E. (2011). Surveying transitional experience and subjective well-being: income, work, family. *Economic Systems*, *35*(2), 139–157.

Self, A., Thomas, J., & Randall, C. (2012). *Measuring national well-being: life in the UK, 2012*. London: Office for National Statistics.

Seligman, M. (1975). *Helplessness. On depression, development, and death*. New York: W H Freeman and co.

Seligman, M. E., Steen, T. A., Park, N., & Peterson, C. (2005). Positive psychology progress: empirical validation of interventions. *The American Psychologist*, *60*(5), 410–421. doi: 10.1037/0003-066X.60.5.410

Seligman, M. E. P. (2003). *Authentic happiness: using the new positive psychology to realize your potential for deep fulfillment*. London: Nicholas Brealey.

Seligman, M. E. P. (2011). *Flourish: a new understanding of happiness and well-being – and how to achieve them*. London: Nicholas Brealey Publishing.

Seligman, R. (2005). From affliction to affirmation: narrative transformation and the therapeutics of Candomble mediumship. *Transcultural Psychiatry*, *42*(2), 272–294.

Selye, H. (1998). A syndrome produced by diverse nocuous agents. 1936. *The Journal of Neuropsychiatry and Clinical Neurosciences*, *10*(2), 230–231.

Sergeant, S., & Mongrain, M. (2011). Are positive psychology exercises helpful for people with depressive personality styles? *The Journal of Positive Psychology*, *6*(4), 260–272. doi: 10.1080/17439760.2011.577089

Sharma, R., Gupta, N., & Bijlani, R. L. (2008). Effect of yoga based lifestyle intervention on subjective well-being. *Indian Journal of Physiology and Pharmacology*, *52*(2), 123–131.

Sheridan, M. A., Fox, N. A., Zeanah, C. H., McLaughlin, K. A., & Nelson, C. A. (2012). Variation in neural development as a result of exposure to institutionalization early in childhood. *Proceedings of the National Academy of Sciences*, *109*(32), 12927–12932.

Shonkoff, J. P., & Garner, A. S. (2012). The lifelong effects of early childhood adversity and toxic stress. *Pediatrics*, *129*(1), e232–246. doi: 10.1542/peds.2011-2663

Shryack, J., Steger, M. F., Krueger, R. F., & Kallie, C. S. (2010). The structure of virtue: an empirical investigation of the dimensionality of the virtues in action inventory of strengths. *Personality and Individual Differences*, *48*(6), 714–719. doi: http://dx.doi.org/10.1016/j.paid.2010.01.007

Simon, J., Pilling, S., Burbeck, R., & Goldberg, D. (2006). Treatment options in moderate and severe depression: decision analysis supporting a clinical guideline. *The British Journal of Psychiatry*, *189*(6), 494–501.

Simon, L., Greenberg, J., Harmon-Jones, E., Solomon, S., Pyszczynski, T., Arndt, J., & Abend, T. (1997). Terror management and cognitive-experiential self-theory: evidence that terror management occurs in the experiential system. *Journal Personality and Social Psychology*, *72*(5), 1132–1146.

Singer, J. A., Blagov, P., Berry, M., & Oost, K. M. (2012). Self-defining memories, scripts, and the life story: narrative identity in personality and psychotherapy. *Journal of Personality*. doi: 10.1111/jopy.12005

Singer, P. (2005). Ethics and intuition. *Journal of Ethics*, *9*, 331–352.

Slagboom, P. E., Beekman, M., Passtoors, W. M., Deelen, J., Vaarhorst, A. A. M., Boer, J. M., . . . Westendorp, R. G. J. (2011). Genomics of human longevity. *Philosophical Transactions of the Royal Society B: Biological Sciences*, *366*(1561), 35–42.

Smith, A. S., & Wang, Z. (2012). Salubrious effects of oxytocin on social stress-induced deficits. *Hormones and Behavior*, *61*(3), 320–330. doi: 10.1016/j.yhbeh.2011.11.010

Smith, J. C. (1976). Psychotherapeutic effects of transcendental meditation with controls for expectation of relief and daily sitting. *Journal of Consulting & Clinical Psychology*, *44*, 630–637.

Spinoza, B. de & Wolf, A. (1910). *Short treatise on God, man and his well-being*. [S.l.]. London: Adam and Charles Black.

Starr, J. M., & Deary, I. J. (2011). Socio-economic position predicts grip strength and its decline between 79 and 87 years: the Lothian Birth Cohort 1921. *Age and Ageing*, *40*(6), 749–752. doi: 10.1093/ageing/afr070

Steger, M. F., Kashdan, T. B., & Oishi, S. (2008). Being good by doing good: daily eudaimonic activity and well-being. *Journal of Research in Personality*, *42*(1), 22–42.

Steptoe, A., Demakakos, P., de Oliveira, C., & Wardle, J. (2012). Distinctive biological correlates of positive psychological well-being in older men and women. *Psychosomatic Medicine*, *74*(5), 501–508. doi: 10.1097/PSY.0b013e31824f82c8

Steptoe, A., & Wardle, J. (2011). Positive affect measured using ecological momentary assessment and survival in older men and women. *Proceedings of the National Academy of Sciences*, *108*(45), 18244–18248. doi: 10.1073/pnas.1110892108

Stevenson, J. (1999). The treatment of the long-term sequelae of child abuse. *Journal Of Child Psychology And Psychiatry And Allied Disciplines*, *40*(1), 89–111.

Stiglitz, J., Sen, A., & Fitoussi, J.-P. (2009). Report by the Commission on the Measurement of Economic Performance and Social Progress. Retrieved from www.stiglitz-sen-fitoussi.fr/en/index.htm

Stonington, S. (2011). Facing death, gazing inward: end-of-life and the transformation of clinical subjectivity in Thailand. *Culture, Medicine, and Psychiatry*, *35*(2), 113–133. doi: 10.1007/s11013-011-9210-6

Strobel, M., Tumasjan, A., & Spörrle, M. (2011). Be yourself, believe in yourself, and be happy: self-efficacy as a mediator between personality factors and subjective well-being. *Scandinavian Journal of Psychology*, *52*(1), 43–48. doi: 10.1111/j.1467-9450.2010.00826.x

Stroebe, M., Finkenauer, C., Wijngaards-de Meij, L., Schut, H., van den Bout, J., & Stroebe, W. (2013). Partner-oriented self-regulation among bereaved parents: the costs of holding in grief for the partner's sake. *Psychological Science*, *24*(4), 395–402.

Sugaya, L., Hasin, D. S., Olfson, M., Lin, K. H., Grant, B. F., & Blanco, C. (2012). Child physical abuse and adult mental health: a national study. *Journal of Traumatic Stress*, *25*(4), 384–392. doi: 10.1002/jts.21719

Svenson, U., Nordfjäll, K., Baird, D., Roger, L., Osterman, P., Hellenius, M.-L., & Roos, G. (2011). Blood cell telomere length is a dynamic feature. *PLoS ONE, 6*(6), e21485. doi: 10.1371/journal.pone.0021485

Talbott, W. J. (2010). *Human rights and human well-being*. New York: Oxford University Press.

Tantam, D. (1993). The developmental psychopathology of emotional disorders. *Journal of the Royal Society of Medicine, 86*(6), 336–340.

Tantam, D. (2003). The flavour of emotions. *Psychology and Psychotherapy, 76*(Pt 1), 23–45.

Tantam, D. (2009). *Can the world afford autistic spectrum disorder? Nonverbal communication, asperger syndrome and the interbrain*. London: Jessica Kingsley Publishers.

Tantam, D. (1999). One reason for you, and one for me. The case for new evidential criteria for psychotherapy being needed and what those might be. In C. Mace (Ed.), *Evidence in the Balance*. London: Routledge.

Tavits, M. (2008). Representation, corruption, and subjective well-being. *Comparative Political Studies, 41*(12), 1607–1630.

Teasdale, J. D., Segal, Z. V., Williams, J. M., Ridgeway, V. A., Soulsby, J. M., & Lau, M. A. (2000). Prevention of relapse/recurrence in major depression by mindfulness-based cognitive therapy. *Journal of Consulting Clinical Psychology, 68*(4), 615–623.

Teerawichitchainan, B., & Korinek, K. (2012). The long-term impact of war on health and wellbeing in Northern Vietnam: some glimpses from a recent survey. *Social Science & Medicine, 74*(12), 1995–2004. doi: 10.1016/j.socscimed.2012.01.040

Terracciano, A., Lockenhoff, C. E., Zonderman, A. B., Ferrucci, L., & Costa, P. T., Jr. (2008). Personality predictors of longevity: activity, emotional stability, and conscientiousness. *Psychosomatic Medicine, 70*(6), 621–627. doi: 10.1097/PSY.0b013e31817b9371

Thoits, P. A. (2006). Personal agency in the stress process. *Journal of Health Social Behaviour, 47*(4), 309–323.

Thompson, R. F. (2009). Habituation: a history. *Neurobiology of Learning and Memory, 92*(2), 127–134. doi: 10.1016/j.nlm.2008.07.011

Tobgay, T., Dophu, U., Torres, C. E., & Na-Bangchang, K. (2011). Health and gross national happiness: review of current status in Bhutan. *Journal of Multidisciplinary Healthcare, 4*, 293–298. doi: 10.2147/JMDH.S21095

Trautmann, S. A., Fehr, T., & Herrmann, M. (2009). Emotions in motion: dynamic compared to static facial expressions of disgust and happiness reveal more widespread emotion-specific activations. *Brain Research, 1284*(0), 100–115. doi: 10.1016/j.brainres.2009.05.075

Trentini, C., Wagner, G., Chachamovich, E., Figueiredo, M., da Silva, L., Hirakata, V., & Fleck, M. (2011). Subjective perception of health in elderly inpatients. *International Journal of Psychology*. doi: 10.1080/00207594.2011.626046

Troisi, J. D., & Gabriel, S. (2011). Chicken soup really is good for the soul. *Psychological Science, 22*(6), 747–753.

Tucker-Drob, E. M., Rhemtulla, M., Harden, K. P., Turkheimer, E., & Fask, D. (2011). Emergence of a gene-by-socioeconomic status interaction on infant mental ability between 10 Months and 2 Years. *Psychological Science, 22*(1), 125–133. doi: 10.1177/0956797610392926

Tumminello, M., Miccichè, S., Dominguez, L. J., Lamura, G., Melchiorre, M. G., Barbagallo, M., & Mantegna, R. N. (2011). Happy aged people are all alike, while every unhappy aged person is unhappy in its own way. *PLoS ONE, 6*(9), e23377. doi: 10.1371/journal.pone.0023377

Turner, A. (2010). *The future of finance: the LSE report*. London: London School of Economics & Political Science.

Turney, K. (2012). Pathways of disadvantage: explaining the relationship between maternal depression and children's problem behaviors. *Social Science Research, 41*(6), 1546–1564. doi: 10.1016/j.ssresearch.2012.06.003

Tversky, A., & Kahneman, D. (1974). Judgment under uncertainty: heuristics and biases. *Science, 185*(4157), 1124–1131.

Ura, K., Alkire, S., & Zangmo, T. (2012). Gross national happiness and the GNH index. In J. F. Helliwell, R. Layard & J. Sachs (Eds), *World happiness report*. New York: The Earth Institute, Columbia University.

Van Deurzen, E. (2009). *Psychotherapy and the quest for happiness*. London: SAGE.

van Gelderen, B. R., Bakker, A. B., Konijn, E. A., & Demerouti, E. (2011). Daily suppression of discrete emotions during the work of police service workers and criminal investigation officers. *Anxiety, stress, and coping, 24*(5), 515–537. doi: 10.1080/10615806.2011.560665

Vartanian, O., Navarrete, G., Chatterjee, A., Fich, L. B., Leder, H., Modroño, C., . . . Skov, M. (2013). Impact of contour on aesthetic judgments and approach-avoidance decisions in architecture. *Proceedings of the National Academy of Sciences*.

Ventegodt, S., Andersen, N. J., & Merrick, J. (2003). Quality of life philosophy I. Quality of life, happiness, and meaning in life. *The Scientific World Journal, 3*, 1164–1175. doi: 10.1100/tsw.2003.102

Ventegodt, S., Flensborg-Madsen, T., Andersen, N. J., & Merrick, J. (2006). What influence do major events in life have on our later quality of life? A retrospective study on life events and associated emotions. *Medical Science Monitor, 12*(2), SR9–15.

Verduyn, P., & Brans, K. (2012). The relationship between extraversion, neuroticism and aspects of trait affect. *Personality and Individual Differences, 52*(6), 664–669. doi: 10.1016/j.paid.2011.12.017

Von Neumann, J., & Morgenstern, O. (1953). *Theory of games and economic behavior* (3rd edn). Princeton, NJ: Princeton University Press.

Voos, A. C., Pelphrey, K. A., & Kaiser, M. D. (2012). Autistic traits are associated with diminished neural response to affective touch. *Social Cognitive and Affective Neuroscience*. doi: 10.1093/scan/nss009

Vygotsky, L. (1966). *Thought and language*. Cambridge, MA: Harvard University Press.

Wadsworth, T. (2013). Sex and the pursuit of happiness: how other people's sex lives are related to our sense of well-being. *Social Indicators Research*, 1–21. doi: 10.1007/s11205-013-0267-1

Wagner, D. D., Altman, M., Boswell, R. G., Kelley, W. M., & Heatherton, T. F. (2013). Self-regulatory depletion enhances neural responses to rewards and impairs top-down control. *Psychological Science, 24*(11), 2262–2271. doi: 10.1177/0956797613492985

Walfisch, S., Maoz, B., & Antonovsky, H. (1984). Sexual satisfaction among middle-aged couples: correlation with frequency of intercourse and health status. *Maturitas, 6*(3), 285–296. doi: http://dx.doi.org/10.1016/0378-5122(84)90045-8

Walum, H., Lichtenstein, P., Neiderhiser, J. M., Reiss, D., Ganiban, J. M., Spotts, E. L., . . . Westberg, L. (2012). Variation in the oxytocin receptor gene is associated with pair-bonding and social behavior. *Biological Psychiatry, 71*(5), 419–426. doi: 10.1016/j.biopsych.2011.09.002

Wang, H., Dwyer-Lindgren, L., Lofgren, K. T., Rajaratnam, J. K., Marcus, J. R., Levin-Rector, A., . . . Murray, C. J. L. (2012). Age-specific and sex-specific mortality in 187 countries, 1970-2010: a systematic analysis for the Global Burden of Disease Study 2010. *The Lancet, 380*(9859), 2071–2094.

Wang, N., Kosinski, M., Stillwell, D., & Rust, J. (2014) Can well-being be measured using Facebook status updates? Validation of Facebook's gross national happiness index. *Social Indicators Research*, 1–9. doi: 10.1007/s11205-012-9996-9

Weber, M., Ruch, W., Littman-Ovadia, H., Lavy, S., & Gai, O. (2013). Relationships among higher-order strengths factors, subjective well-being, and general self-efficacy – the case of Israeli adolescents. *Personality and Individual Differences, 55*(3), 322–327. doi: http://dx.doi.org/10.1016/j.paid.2013.03.006

Weiser, E. (2012). Associations between positive and negative affect and 12-month physical disorders in a national sample. *Journal of Clinical Psychology in Medical Settings, 19*(2), 197–210. doi: 10.1007/s10880-011-9277-9

Weisman, O., Zagoory-Sharon, O., & Feldman, R. (2012). Oxytocin administration to parent enhances infant physiological and behavioral readiness for social engagement. *Biological Psychiatry*. doi: 10.1016/j.biopsych.2012.06.011

Weiss, A., Adams, M. J., & King, J. E. (2011). Happy orang-utans live longer lives. *Biology Letters, 7*(6), 872–874. doi: 10.1098/rsbl.2011.0543

Weiss, R. (1973). *The experience of emotional and social isolation*. Cambridge, MA: MIT Press.

Westermeyer, J. F. (2013). Predictors and characteristics of successful aging among men: a 48-year longitudinal study. *International Journal of Aging & Human Development, 76*(4), 323–345.

Whisman, M. A., & Baucom, D. H. (2012). Intimate relationships and psychopathology. *Clinical Child and Family Psychology Review, 15*(1), 4–13. doi: 10.1007/s10567-011-0107-2

Whissell, T. (1991). Phonoemotional profiling: a description of the emotional flavour of English texts on the basis of the phonemes employed in them. *Perceptual and Motor Skills, 2000*(Oct.), 617–648.

Whitton, S. W., & Kuryluk, A. D. (2012). Relationship satisfaction and depressive symptoms in emerging adults: cross-sectional associations and moderating effects of relationship characteristics. *Journal of Family Psychology: JFP: Journal of the Division of Family Psychology of the American Psychological Association, 26*(2), 226–235. doi: 10.1037/a0027267

WHO ([1946] 2006). Preamble to the Constitution of the World Health Organization as adopted by the International Health Conference, New York, 19–22 June, 1946; signed on 22 July 1946 by the representatives of 61 States (Official Records of the World Health Organization, no. 2, p. 100) and entered into force on 7 April 1948. New York: International Health Conference. Reproduced in WHO (2006). *Basic Documents* (45th edn). Geneva: World Health Organization.

Wiest, M., Schüz, B., & Wurm, S. (2013). Life satisfaction and feeling in control: indicators of successful aging predict mortality in old age. *Journal of Health Psychology, 18*(9), 1199–1208.

Wilhelm, T., & Andress, J. (2011). Psychological weaknesses. In *Ninja Hacking* (pp. 151–165). Boston, MA: Syngress.

Wilkinson, R. G., & Pickett, K. (2010). *The spirit level: why equality is better for everyone* (New edn). London: Penguin.

Willcox, D. C., Willcox, B. J., Todoriki, H., & Suzuki, M. (2009). The Okinawan diet: health implications of a low-calorie, nutrient-dense, antioxidant-rich dietary pattern low in glycemic load. *The Journal of the American College of Nutrition, 28 Suppl*, 500S–516S.

Williams, J. M. (2010). Commentary: mindfulness and psychological process. *Emotion, 10*, 1–7.

Wilt, J., Noftle, E. E., Fleeson, W., & Spain, J. S. (2012). The dynamic role of personality states in mediating the relationship between extraversion and positive affect. *The Journal of Personality, 80*(5), 1205–1236. doi: 10.1111/j.1467-6494.2011.00756.x

Winefield, H. R., & Cormack, S. M. (1986). Regular activities as indicators of subjective health status. *International Journal of Rehabilitation Research, 9*(1), 47–52.

Wittgenstein, L. (1958). *Philosophical investigations* (2nd Vol.). Oxford: Basil Blackwell.

Wnuk, M., & Marcinkowski, J. T. (2012). Do existential variables mediate between religious-spiritual facets of functionality and psychological wellbeing. *Journal of Religion and Health*. doi: 10.1007/s10943-012-9597-6

Woloski-Wruble, A. C., Oliel, Y., Leefsma, M., & Hochner-Celnikier, D. (2010). Sexual activities, sexual and life satisfaction, and successful aging in women. *J Sex Med, 7*(7), 2401–2410. doi: 10.1111/j.1743-6109.2010.01747.x

Wolsko, C., Lardon, C., Mohatt, G. V., & Orr, E. (2007). Stress, coping, and well-being among the Yup'ik of the Yukon-Kuskokwim Delta: the role of enculturation and acculturation. *International Journal of Circumpolar Health, 66*(1), 51–61.

Wood, A. M., & Tarrier, N. (2010). Positive clinical psychology: a new vision and strategy for integrated research and practice. *Clinical Psychology Review, 30*(7), 819–829. doi: 10.1016/j.cpr.2010.06.003

Wood, A. M., Joseph, S., & Maltby, J. (2008). Gratitude uniquely predicts satisfaction with life: incremental validity above the domains and facets of the five factor model. *Personality and Individual Differences, 45*(1), 49–54. doi: 10.1016/j.paid.2008.02.019

Yamasue, H., Yee, J. R., Hurlemann, R., Rilling, J. K., Chen, F. S., Meyer-Lindenberg, A., & Tost, H. (2012). Integrative approaches utilizing oxytocin to enhance prosocial behavior: from animal and human social behavior to autistic social dysfunction. *The Journal of Neuroscience: the official journal of the Society for Neuroscience, 32*(41), 14109–14117. doi: 10.1523/JNEUROSCI.3327-12.2012

Zelenski, J., Santoro, M., & Whelan, D. (2012). Would introverts be better off if they acted more like extraverts? Exploring emotional and cognitive consequences of counterdispositional behavior. *Emotion, 12*(2), 290–303. doi: 10.1037/a0025169

Zhai, Q., Willis, M., O'Shea, B., Zhai, Y., & Yang, Y. (2012). Big Five personality traits, job satisfaction and subjective wellbeing in China. *International Journal of Psychology: Journal international de psychologie*. doi: 10.1080/00207594.2012.732700

Zheng, D., Macera, C. A., Croft, J. B., Giles, W. H., Davis, D., & Scott, W. K. (1997). Major depression and all-cause mortality among white adults in the United States. *Annals of Epidemiology, 7*(3), 213–218.

Zheng, Y., & Cleveland, H. H. (2013). Identifying gender-specific developmental trajectories of nonviolent and violent delinquency from adolescence to young adulthood. *Journal of Adolescence, 36*(2), 371–381. doi: http://dx.doi.org/10.1016/j.adolescence.2012.12.007

Index